Cardiovascular Reactivity and Stress

Patterns of Physiological Response

J. Rick Turner

University of Tennessee
Memphis, Tennessee

Plenum Press • New York and London

Library of Congress Cataloging-in-Publication Data

Turner, J. Rick.
    Cardiovascular reactivity and stress : patterns of physiological
response / J. Rick Turner.
       p.   cm. -- (Plenum series in behavioral psychophysiology and
    medicine)
    Includes bibliographical references and index.
    ISBN 0-306-44612-X
    1. Heart--Diseases--Psychosomatic aspect. 2. Heart-
-Psychophysiology. 3. Stress (Psychology)   I. Title. II. Series.
    [DNLM: 1. Cardiovascular System--physiology. 2. Stress,
Psychological--physiopathology. 3. Hypertension--etiology.   WG 102
T948c 1994]
RC682.9.T87   1994
616.1'08--dc20
DNLM/DLC
for Library of Congress   93-43748
                                                             CIP

Coventry University

ISBN 0-306-44612-X

©1994 Plenum Press, New York
A Division of Plenum Publishing Corporation
233 Spring Street, New York, N.Y. 10013

Printed in the United States of America

Cardiovascular Reactivity and Stress

Patterns of Physiological Response

THE PLENUM SERIES IN BEHAVIORAL PSYCHOPHYSIOLOGY AND MEDICINE

Series Editor:
William J. Ray, *Pennsylvania State University, University Park, Pennsylvania*

BIOLOGICAL BARRIERS IN BEHAVIORAL MEDICINE
  Edited by Wolfgang Linden

CARDIOVASCULAR REACTIVITY AND STRESS
Patterns of Physiological Response
  J. Rick Turner

CLINICAL APPLIED PSYCHOPHYSIOLOGY
  Edited by John G. Carlson, A. Ronald Seifert, and Niels Birbaumer

ELECTRODERMAL ACTIVITY
  Wolfram Boucsein

HANDBOOK OF RESEARCH METHODS IN CARDIOVASCULAR
BEHAVIORAL MEDICINE
  Edited by Neil Schneiderman, Stephen M. Weiss,
  and Peter G. Kaufmann

INTERNATIONAL PERSPECTIVES ON SELF-REGULATION AND
HEALTH
  Edited by John G. Carlson and A. Ronald Seifert

PHYSIOLOGY AND BEHAVIOR THERAPY
Conceptual Guidelines for the Clinician
  James G. Hollandsworth, Jr.

THE PHYSIOLOGY OF PSYCHOLOGICAL DISORDERS
Schizophrenia, Depression, Anxiety, and Substance Abuse
  James G. Hollandsworth, Jr.

THE PSYCHOLOGY AND PHYSIOLOGY OF BREATHING
In Behavioral Medicine, Clinical Psychology, and Psychiatry
  Robert Fried with Joseph Grimaldi

SOCIAL SUPPORT AND CARDIOVASCULAR DISEASE
  Edited by Sally A. Shumaker and Susan M. Czajkowski

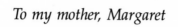

To my mother, Margaret

Foreword

This book is an articulate, concise, contemporary introduction to the study of important variables underlying cardiovascular reactivity. Its strength is in the combination of a scholarly but nonpedantic approach to cardiovascular psychophysiology and a solid understanding of behavioral medicine approaches to the study of hypertension. The topics covered are central to the study of relationships between behavior and cardiovascular reactivity; the list of suggested readings at the end of each chapter provides excellent guidance for more detailed study of specific issues.

It has now been more than a dozen years since Plenum Press published Paul Obrist's seminal monograph *Cardiovascular Psychophysiology*. The volume had a major impact in relating cardiovascular regulation to behaving individuals and in developing thoughtful hypotheses concerning such factors as they might pertain to hypertension. The impact of that work extended across scientific disciplines as well as aross continents. At the time the Obrist book was published, a young psychologist, J. Rick Turner, was completing his Ph.D. thesis in psychology at the University of Birmingham, England, on heart rate reactions to psychological challenge. After continued collaboration for the next several years with his former Ph.D. mentor, Douglas Carroll, Turner joined the Obrist laboratory at the University of North Carolina. Although Obrist unfortunately died during Turner's tenure in the laboratory, collaboration continued with Kathleen Light and Andrew Sherwood. The enlightened legacy of the North Carolina laboratory can clearly be seen in this text.

A central hypothesis discussed in the volume is that cardiovascular reactivity may be a risk factor for essential hypertension. Turner carefully points out that the potential link between elevated cardiovascular reactivity and cardiovascular disease may occur either as a marker of risk or as a causal mechanism. In either case it would be important from the standpoint of predicting later disease. As a trained methodologist, however, Turner emphasizes that the extent to which cardiovascular reactivity can be considered as a risk factor in part involves demonstrating that it provides a stable measure of individual differences. In a well-balanced, thoughtful review of this issue, Turner describes strong evidence of temporal stability for cardiovascular reactivity and discusses important issues concerning intertask consistency and laboratory-to-field generalization.

The major strengths of the book are in providing a balanced evaluation of the phenomenon of cardiovascular reactivity and in offering valuable insights into its potential links with hypertension. Although biomedical scientists primarily interested in hypertension might wish to know more about how reactivity is linked to distribution of the blood flow in low-flow circulatory states, the role of central nervous system drive in the regulation of pressure or flow, sensitization of receptors by sodium, possible subcategories of essential hypertension, or the role of insulin metabolism in sympathetic nervous system activity and sodium retention, Turner wisely restricts his discussion to those issues in which behavioral medicine research has facilitated an understanding of cardiovascular reactivity. The discussions in the present volume concerning age, ethnicity, gender, personality, and renal factors as contributors to individual differences in reactivity are valuable. So too is the fascinating chapter on genetic determinants of individual differences in reactivity.

In summary, this text provides a valuable introduction to the study of cardiovascular reactivity and its importance in behavioral medicine research. The evidence that cardiovascular reactivity may be a risk factor for cardiovascular disease is provocative and potentially important. This book is written at a level that should permit behavioral scientists without extensive biomedical training to understand in detail the role that cardiovascular reactivity may play as a risk factor for cardiovascular disease. Conversely, it is sufficiently scholarly and well-written to provide critical insights to biomedical scientists who may be intrigued by potential relationships between behavior and cardiovascular disease. It is certainly a timely, important, and valuable book.

NEIL SCHNEIDERMAN
James L. Knight Professor of Psychology,
  Psychiatry, Medicine, and
  Biomedical Engineering
University of Miami
Coral Gables, Florida

Preface

Cardiovascular reactivity refers to changes in cardiovascular activity associated primarily with exposure to psychological stress. The investigation of reactivity is of considerable interest to scientists from the disciplines of psychology, psychosomatic medicine, and behavioral medicine. Psychologists are particularly interested in it because different individuals show different amounts of reactivity under the same conditions. This individual variation has led reactivity to be regarded as an individual difference dimension, and all individual difference phenomena are of interest to psychologists. However, reactivity has also attracted additional experimental attention because of hypothesized links between sizable stress responses and the later development of cardiovascular disease. Researchers from the fields of psychosomatic and behavioral medicine have therefore extensively investigated the characteristics of reactivity. This volume introduces and discusses some of the experiments that have examined these characteristics and places them within a behavioral medicine/psychosomatic medicine framework.

Behavioral medicine and psychosomatic medicine are interdisciplinary fields that investigate the role of behavior in the development of disease. They are concerned with mechanisms of behavioral influence, prevention, detection, treatment, and rehabilitation. Medical doctors, psychologists, health educators, and many other health professionals work together to use behavioral science in these pursuits. Cardiovascular behavioral medicine is the subdiscipline of behavioral medicine that focuses on behavioral influences in cardiovascular disorders. In this volume we shall concentrate on one particular disorder—hypertension.

Hypertension, or high blood pressure, is an extremely prevalent disease in industrialized societies. It is also of added significance because it is a potent risk factor for coronary heart disease, which is responsible for more adult deaths in Western countries than any other single cause.

The following chapters investigate the occurrence and nature of cardiovascular reactivity and describe the relationships among stress, reactivity, and potential disease outcomes. The text is divided into three parts. The first part provides an introduction to the cardiovascular system, its control by the nervous system, and the laboratory elicitation and assessment of reactivity. Potential links between large cardiovascular stress responses and the later development of hypertension are also discussed. The second part describes laboratory experiments designed to explore both individual and group differences in reactivity. The relationship between cardiovascular activity during stress and concurrent metabolic needs is explored, and the influence of genetic inheritance is investigated. Finally, the third part starts with an overview of studies that have explored cardiovascular activity during naturally occurring stressful situations encountered during everyday activities. Although laboratory investigation of reactivity is extremely useful because of the tight experimental control that is possible, investigation of stress responses during natural circumstances is crucial. If reactivity does play a role in the development of cardiovascular disease, it is in the presence of everyday stressors that these reactions will take their toll. The penultimate chapter explores the topic of risk determination, and it considers whether it might be possible to develop an information-gathering protocol that will enable the identification of young people at risk for the later development of cardiovascular disease. If this can be done successfully, the final chapter observes, intervention strategies become a possibility. Detailed discussion of such strategies is beyond the focus of this volume, but references are provided to point the reader in appropriate directions.

While writing this volume, I have tried to keep two categories of potential readers in mind. Various aspects of the text's organization will, I hope, make the contents accessible and informative to each type of reader. First, for the reader who is simply interested in learning something about reactivity, I have tried to provide a self-contained introduction to the topic. Reading the chapters sequentially should provide some idea of what reactivity research is about without necessitating referral to other sources. Second, for students who wish to become more thoroughly acquainted with the topic, lists of further readings are provided at the end of each chapter. These readings, along with the references at the end of the volume, should provide starting points for further study. The readings can be pursued by individual students or by members of a class. Small groups of students may wish to study one reading each and report back to the class as a whole; discussions of this material may prove particularly helpful.

Of course, only the reader can evaluate whether I have achieved my goals. I should be pleased to receive feedback on any aspect of how the volume might be improved. I can be contacted at the Division of Pediatric Cardiology, Department of Pediatrics, College of Medicine, University of Tennessee, Memphis, 777 Washington Avenue, Suite 215, Memphis, TN 38105.

Many people have provided personal and professional support that contributed to the completion of this project. Thanks are expressed to Robert Brown, Michael Byng, Douglas Carroll, Raymond Cochrane, David and Ian Crowley, Barbara Dodd, Clive Eastman, John Hewitt, Lisa Jack, Roy Jeans, Donna Lang, Lynn Liben, Kathleen Light, Lia Marini, Robert Mears, Graham Millard, Nancy Norvell, David Ragland, Robert Stern, Julian Thayer, and Marcia Ward. Thanks also to Gary Swan of SRI International, who allowed me to access SRI's Health Sciences library facilities, and to many authors who sent me reprints and preprints. While many authors have written eloquently on the topic of reactivity, I have found particular inspiration in the work of Stephen Manuck and the late Paul Obrist.

Eliot Werner at Plenum, at whose invitation this project was undertaken, and series editor William Ray provided essential help throughout all stages of the book's development. Much needed feedback on earlier drafts was given by John Hewitt, Kathleen Light, William Lovallo, James McCubbin, and Andrew Sherwood. While it is almost unfair to single out one of these readers, I should like to acknowledge that Bill Lovallo provided extensive and detailed advice concerning the content and structure of two chapters I found particularly hard to write; special thanks are accordingly expressed to him.

The original manuscript was prepared by Dot Faulkner, Donna Taylor, and Pat Taylor; thanks are expressed to them, and to Jocelyn Sharlet and Dan Kulkosky at Plenum for production of the published volume.

This text was written while I was supported by a National Heart, Lung and Blood Institutional Research Training Grant (T32 HL07365), granted to the School of Public Health, University of California, Berkeley. I am indebted to David Ragland, the training program director, for giving me the academic freedom to pursue this project.

Finally, I thank my friend and colleague Andrew Sherwood for his immeasurable help during the past ten years. He has shared his ideas and expertise generously and selflessly, and his scholarly insights have profoundly influenced my thinking. I have no doubt that without his help, I could not have written this book.

J. RICK TURNER

Memphis, Tennessee

Contents

PART I

Orientation: Concepts, Systems, and Methods

CHAPTER 1

Cardiovascular Reactivity and Stress: Introduction and Overview

Cardiovascular reactivity research examines the alterations in cardiovascular activity that occur in response to environmental circumstances considered to be stressful. These circumstances are often discrete, identifiable stressors (such as short experimental tasks), but they can also be more long-lasting (such as a period of hours spent at work). *Reactivity* refers to a change in activity. As an example, consider heart rate reactivity. Its calculation requires a measure of heart rate during an unstressed period (often called a *baseline* period) and a measure of heart rate during the stressor. The easiest way of calculating reactivity, which has recently received renewed endorsement (Llabre *et al.*, 1991; Pickering, 1991b), is to subtract the baseline level from the level of activity during the stressor. Thus, if one's heart rate is 70 beats per minute (bpm) during the unstressed period and 100 bpm during the stressor, one's reactivity score on this occasion would be 30 bpm. More rigorous description and definitions of reactivity will follow in later chapters.

An interesting observation concerning cardiovascular reactivity is that there is considerable variation in the amount of reactivity displayed by different individuals in the same situation. One person may show very little reactivity while another person may have a heart rate reactivity score of 40 or 50 bpm. This individual variation in cardiovascular responses to psychological stress has led to the conceptualization of reactivity as an individual differences dimension (Manuck *et al.*, 1989). These individual differences are fascinating in their own right, and, like all individual difference phenomena, are of intrinsic interest to experi-

3

mental psychologists. However, it is important to note here that individual variation in cardiovascular reactivity has attracted additional experimental attention because of hypothesized links between large stress responses and the later development of cardiovascular disease (Turner et al., 1992). Scientists from the disciplines of psychophysiology, psychosomatic medicine, and behavioral medicine have conducted many studies examining various aspects of cardiovascular reactivity. This research is introduced in the following chapters.

Psychophysiology

Psychophysiology is the division of psychology that investigates changes in the activity of physiological systems caused by psychological input. A more thorough definition was provided by Andreassi (1989), who defined psychophysiology as "the study of relations between psychological manipulations and resulting physiological responses, measured in the living organism, to promote understanding of the relation between mental and bodily processes." The relationship between mental and bodily processes, though viewed and expressed differently at different times, has been of interest to philosophers and scientists for thousands of years, and psychophysiology continues in this tradition. In modern terminology, the changes in physiological activity caused by psychological stressors can be expressed as psychophysiological reactivity.

The psychophysiological strategy has been employed extensively in the investigation of reactivity. This strategy includes the development of electronic equipment to facilitate highly sophisticated measurement of physiological activity, and the rigorous testing of hypotheses via appropriate experimental designs. In this manner, the psychophysiological strategy provides fundamental knowledge concerning the interaction of mental and bodily processes (Andreassi, 1989). This strategy has been employed in the fields of psychosomatic medicine and behavioral medicine to investigate hypothesized links between reactivity and cardiovascular disease.

Psychosomatic Medicine

The development of psychosomatic medicine, which can to some extent be viewed as a forerunner of behavioral medicine, was closely allied to the prominence at that time of Freud's psychoanalytic theory. An increasing interest in the interplay between emotional events and physiological activity led the National Research Council to begin publishing the journal *Psychosomatic Medicine* in 1939. In 1943, this field became organized into a society, now called the American Psychosomatic Society. Influential early leaders were primarily psychiatrists and psychodynamically oriented psychologists, and interest often focused on psychoanalytical interpretations of health problems such as ulcers, asthma, and high blood pressure. These disorders represented a group of disorders that could not be neatly slotted into any of the categories of disorders in the biomedical model, which was a dominant force in medicine during the nineteenth century and early years of the twentieth century.

The biomedical model proposed that all diseases or physical disorders could be explained by disturbances in physiological patterns resulting from injury, biochemical imbalances, or bacterial and viral infections. The group of disorders such as ulcers, asthma, and high blood pressure could not be explained in this way. They were classified as nervous conditions, and a complaint of nervous origin was understood as having no physical basis.

These various disorders are now referred to as *psychosomatic disorders*. The word *psychosomatic* is derived from "psyche" (mind) and "soma" (body) and refers to their interaction. Despite this derivation of the word psychosomatic, many scientists would now agree that the two aspects (mind and body) are totally interdependent in terms of both functional effects and health.

Psychosomatic theory, then, historically viewed some somatic complaints as primarily caused by unconscious psychological conflicts. High blood pressure, a condition referred to as *hypertension*, was believed to be the result of a conflict between feelings of anger and hostility, of which the individual may have been unaware, and a fear of the consequences of expressing these feelings. Because these proposed psychological conflicts are not readily testable in modern scientific ways, the focus of attention in psychosomatic medicine has shifted. Psychosomatic medicine is now a broader field, concerned with the interrelationships between psychological and social factors, biological and physiological functions, and the development and course of illness. However, some modern reactivity studies, such as those exploring the relationship between reactivity and hostility (e.g., Suarez & Williams, 1990; see also T. W. Smith, 1992), demonstrate a clear lineage between old and new psychosomatic medicine.

Behavioral Medicine

The field of behavioral medicine emerged in the 1970s to study the role of behavioral factors in illness. Because behavioral medicine grew out of psychology, the word *behavior* is used here in its broadest sense, including both motor acts and mental activities. A useful definition of behavioral medicine was provided by Schwartz and Weiss (1978) as "the *interdisciplinary* field concerned with the development and *integration* of behavioral *and* medical science knowledge and techniques relevant to health and illness, and the application of this knowledge and these techniques to prevention, diagnosis, treatment and rehabilitation" (p. 250). Behavioral medicine is a wide field of investigation, with an emphasis on interdisciplinary collaboration. Psychologists, sociologists, and various medical specialists (such as epidemiologists and cardiologists) are working together on health issues that are of concern to all these individual disciplines. The Society of Behavioral Medicine was founded in 1979, and its annual meetings attract a large and varied body of participants.

Similarities between Psychosomatic Medicine and Behavioral Medicine

It is true that psychosomatic medicine and behavioral medicine do contain some aspects that reflect their different origins in psychiatry and psychology, respectively. For example, consultation-liaison psychiatry is a core element of psychosomatic medicine, whereas behavioral interventions based on learning theory (e.g., biofeedback; see Birk, 1973) are closely allied to behavioral medicine. Behavioral medicine is also concerned with the health implications of such behaviors as eating inappropriately, using alcohol and nicotine, and engaging in behaviors likely to spread the AIDS virus.

Nevertheless, it is also true that these two disciplines have very similar aspects. From the perspective of this text, their similarities are much more salient than their differences. Both disciplines are interested in mind-body interactions, the mechanisms behind such interactions, and the implications of these interactions for disease and, equally important, for health. Many scientists are members of the American Psychosomatic Society and the Society of Behavioral Medicine, and leading research in cardiovascular stress psychophysiology is presented at both societies' annual meetings.

Behavioral Health and Health Psychology

Two other fields of scientific investigation should also be mentioned here, namely behavioral health and health psychology. Gatchel, Baum, and Krantz (1989) recently discussed the definitions of behavioral medicine, behavioral health, and health psychology proposed by Matarazzo (1980). Matarazzo suggested that, whereas *behavioral medicine* is concerned with health, illness, and related physiological dysfunctions, *behavioral health* is a term describing the interdisciplinary subspeciality within behavioral medicine that focuses specifically on the maintenance of health and the prevention of illness in currently healthy individuals. *Health psychology* is then defined as a more discipline-specific term referring to the role of psychology as a science and a profession in the domains of behavioral medicine and behavioral health (see Matarazzo, 1980).

Overview of This Volume

This text presents an introduction to cardiovascular reactivity research within a behavioral medicine/psychosomatic medicine perspective. Two main areas of cardiovascular behavioral medicine research are hypertension and coronary heart disease. While these two topics share some common ground, description of research addressing them is often presented separately. We shall consider only hypertension in this volume because the majority of research in human subjects exploring links between cardiovascular reactivity and disease has focused on the disease of hypertension. In reality, hypertension and coronary heart disease are closely linked by the fact that hypertension is a powerful risk factor for the development of coronary heart disease. Readers interesting in pursuing behavioral approaches to coronary heart disease are directed to the recent volume by T. W. Smith and Leon (1992).

It should also be made clear at this point that this volume focuses on the first part of Schwartz and Weiss's definition of behavioral medicine—the development and integration of behavioral and biomedical science, knowledge, and techniques relevant to disease. We shall see how the techniques of cardiovascular psychophysiology can be combined with the experimental paradigms of behavioral medicine and psychosomatic medicine to provide a comprehensive description of individual differences in cardiovascular reactivity, and how large cardiovascular responses during stress may be associated with the disease of hypertension.

Experimental Tasks That Elicit Reactivity

Many of the experimental tasks discussed in this volume are designed to be mentally stressful. One example is mental arithmetic. Experimental subjects are asked to perform a mental arithmetic task for several minutes. Such stressors induce psychological activation that in turn elicits cardiovascular changes. Much of our attention will focus on psychological stressors, but the study of reactivity during other tasks should not be minimized. Physical exercise tasks and a stressor known as the *cold pressor* (which involves placing one's hand or foot in ice water) are also used in behavioral medicine paradigms.

Cardiovascular reactivity can be studied in an experimental laboratory using such stressors. A standard stressor, or a group of them, is chosen and each subject in an experiment is presented with the same one. Cardiovascular activity is monitored throughout the study, and subsequent calculation of reactivity scores is performed. Reactivity can also be studied outside the laboratory by employing portable recording devices called *ambulatory monitors*. This procedure, referred to as ambulatory monitoring, is extremely important since it allows us to see how people's cardiovascular systems respond to environmental stressors that occur during everyday activities.

Hypothesized Links between Reactivity and Hypertension

A central hypothesis in this research field is called the *reactivity hypothesis*. In its broadest definition, the reactivity hypothesis suggests that greater cardiovascular reactivity to behavioral stressors may play some role in the development of sustained arterial hypertension (Light et al., 1992b). High reactivity during stressors may therefore be a predictor of later hypertension development. Another relevant possibility is that while high reactivity might not actually play a causal role in the development of hypertension, it is in some way associated with the disease, and accordingly it can be seen in individuals who are at risk for hypertension development. It is important to note that the predictive significance of this second possibility is the same as that for the reactivity hypothesis itself. If reactivity is found to be a good predictor of disease development, this is a very useful observation whether or not the high reactivity actually causes the progression of the disease.

What evidence do we have for believing there might be an association between reactivity and disease? Chapter 4 will address this question in due course, but it is appropriate to summarize some evidence here. First, the cardiovascular changes seen in reactivity during psychological stressors resemble the pattern of cardiovascular activity seen in the condition known as *borderline hypertension*. This condition, which is characterized by mildly elevated blood pressure, is an acknowledged precursor of hypertension. Second, borderline hypertensives show greater reactivity to psychological stressors than do normotensive subjects. Third, individuals who are at acknowledged risk for hypertension because their parents are hypertensive show greater reactivity than do individuals whose parents display normal blood pressure. It must be admitted that none of these lines of evidence provides conclusive proof by itself. However, taken together they are sufficiently persuasive to merit further investigation of this possible link.

Hypertension is a disease of major proportions, affecting 60 million individuals in the United States alone (Kannel & Thom, 1986). All avenues of inquiry that might lead to improved knowledge of the mechanisms of disease development are therefore important to pursue. Accordingly, the chapters that follow report research conducted to examine the phenomenon of cardiovascular reactivity and the possible association between reactivity and hypertension.

Chapter 2 provides an introduction to three physiological systems involved in cardiovascular reactivity. The cardiovascular system is obviously of interest, but it is also important to consider the nervous system and the endocrine system. Both of these systems are involved in initiating the cardiovascular changes seen during stress. Chapter 3 then introduces a range of topics that are important in reactivity research. Key concepts are explained, and several experimental tasks and methodologies are described. A more detailed discussion of the possible links between reactivity and hypertension follows in Chapter 4.

The second section of this text focuses on laboratory investigation of reactivity. Both individual and group differences in reactivity are discussed. Chapter 5 deals with individual differences and documents the considerable individual variation that occurs in response to psychological stressors. The metabolic relevance of cardiac adjustments during such tasks is the focus of Chapter 6. Psychological stressors cause increases in cardiac activity that are different in one important way from those seen during physical labor. During physical labor, when the energy demands (and hence oxygen demands) of the body increase, the heart increases its activity to provide muscles with the necessary extra oxygenated blood. During the psychological stressors discussed in this volume, cardiac increases are seen in the context of very small metabolic demands; the tasks are carefully designed to require very little physical activity. The large cardiac increases shown by certain individuals during these stressors are therefore metabolically excessive, and it is precisely these types of cardiac increases that are actually involved in the hypotheses linking reactivity with disease development.

Next, Chapter 7 examines genetic and environmental influences in the determination of individual differences in cardiovascular responses during psychological stressors. Finally, Chapter 8 looks at group differences in reactivity, examining the influences of age, gender, and race. The influences of personality characteristics and aerobic fitness are also examined, and consideration is given to renal influences on reactivity.

In Part III of the volume, Chapter 9 takes us from the experimental laboratory into the real world. The use of ambulatory monitoring to explore people's responses to naturally occurring stressors is discussed, and the relationship between laboratory and real-world stress responses is examined. Chapter 10 then explores the possible use of reactivity testing, in conjunction with other information-gathering strategies, in the prediction of risk for hypertension development. Such prediction is an extremely important consideration, since successful prediction of risk at an early age would allow us to consider the possibilities of intervention aimed at reducing the chances of actually developing the disease in later life.

Evaluation of the possibility of using reactivity information in successful risk prediction has yet to be achieved, and simply raising this possibility, in one sense, is the culmination of the discussions in the present volume. Full consideration of the topic of intervention is therefore beyond the scope of this volume. However, Chapter 11, the concluding chapter, briefly provides examples of such intervention and also mentions other topics in reactivity research that have not been discussed. In this way, the reader is given some starting directions for pursuing further topics of particular interest.

Further Reading

1. Alexander, F. (1950). *Psychosomatic medicine*. New York: W.W. Norton.
2. Andreassi, J.L. (1989). *Psychophysiology: Human behavior and physiological response* (2nd ed.). Hillsdale, NJ: Erlbaum.
3. Cacioppo, J.T., & Petty, R.E. (1982). *Perspectives in cardiovascular psychophysiology*. New York: Guilford.
4. Coles, M.G.H., Donchin, E., & Porges, S.W. (1986). *Psychophysiology: Systems, processes, and applications*. New York: Guilford.
5. Engel, G.L. (1977). The need for a new medical model: A challenge for biomedicine. *Science, 19B*, 129–136.
6. Garfield, S.L. (Ed.). (1982). Behavioral medicine [Special issue]. *Journal of Consulting and Clinical Psychology, 50*(6).
7. Martin, I., & Venables, P.H. (1980). *Techniques in psychophysiology*. Chichester: Wiley.
8. Obrist, P.A. (1981). *Cardiovascular psychophysiology: A perspective*. New York: Plenum.
9. Obrist, P.A., Black, A.H., Brener, J., & DiCara, L.V. (1974). *Cardiovascular psychophysiology*. Chicago: Aldine.
10. Orlebeke, J.F., Mulder, G., & van Doornen, L.J.P. (1985). *Psychophysiology of cardiovascular control: Methods, models, and data*. New York: Plenum.
11. Pattishall, E.G., Jr. (1989). The development of behavioral medicine: Historical models. *Annals of Behavioral Medicine, 11*, 43–48.
12. Schneiderman, N., Weiss, S.M., & Kaufmann, P.G. (1989). *Handbook of research methods in cardiovascular behavioral medicine*. New York: Plenum.
13. Smith, T.W., & Leon, A.S. (1992). *Coronary heart disease: A behavioral perspective*. Champaign, IL: Research Press.
14. Stern, R.M., Ray, W.J., & Davis, C.M. (1980). *Psychophysiological recording*. New York: Oxford University Press.
15. Weiner, H. (1992). Specificity and specification: Two continuing problems in psychosomatic research. *Psychosomatic Medicine, 54*, 567–587.

CHAPTER 2

The Nervous, Endocrine, and Cardiovascular Systems

Throughout this volume we are concerned with activity and reactivity in the cardiovascular system during psychological stressors. Cardiovascular activity is mediated by the nervous and endocrine systems. Accordingly, we shall now examine the necessary details of each system, and also look at how they interact to produce the cardiovascular responses that are the topic of this text. It should be acknowledged that some aspects of the organization of this chapter are based on that used by Rushmer (1989) in his description of the structure and function of the cardiovascular system, and the reader is referred to his work for further details.

The Nervous System

The nervous system collects information about the state of affairs both within and outside the body, and it responds appropriately. There are, therefore, three main phases in its operation: data collection, data analysis, and action. The nervous system acts like many decision-making organizations dealing with input, information processing, and output.

Figure 2.1 shows how the nervous system is usually described. The two parts of the central nervous system, the brain and the spinal cord, are encased within structures made of bone for protection (the skull and the spinal column, respectively). The central nervous system is the

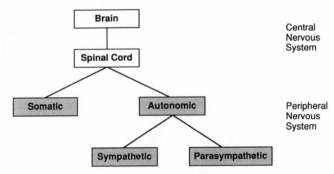

Figure 2.1. A schematic diagram of the human nervous system. The central nervous system (the central command operations center) and the peripheral nervous system (the remainder of the nervous system) are shown. While all aspects of the nervous system are important, this volume will focus in particular upon the sympathetic branch of the autonomic nervous system and its control by the central nervous system during stress.

central command operations center; executive decisions, based upon information gathered elsewhere and relayed here, are made by this system. The peripheral nervous system comprises the remainder of the nervous system.

The sensory nervous system transmits data gathered by the senses to the central nervous system, and the somatic (skeletal) system conveys instructions from the central system to muscles that move the skeleton (i.e., the muscles normally under voluntary control). The autonomic nervous system, on the other hand, can be thought of as being in charge of the basic survival functions of the body that are normally under involuntary control. This includes the operation of the lungs, stomach, kidneys, and the heart. We do not have to tell ourselves to breathe, or tell our heart to beat. It is true that it is possible to "override" the central command center and breathe in a certain pattern, and with somewhat more difficulty (and training in biofeedback), it is possible to exert some conscious influence on heart rate. However, under normal circumstances, we do not have to exert conscious effort in times of stress to tell our heart what to do. All we have to do is to perceive a situation as challenging, and the autonomic system does the rest. Of course, perception itself is also performed by the nervous system.

The last division shown in Figure 2.1 concerns the separation of the autonomic nervous system into sympathetic and parasympathetic branches. The simplest view of these branches is to regard the sympathetic division as being concerned with the mobilization of the body for action, while the parasympathetic division is concerned with calming the body, absorbing nutrients, and conserving energy. These two divisions, therefore, often create opposite effects. The heart, like many organs, is dually innervated by these two divisions of the autonomic nervous system, which means that its activity is the net result of two opposing influences. Increasing sympathetic influence (also called *drive* or *tone*) on the heart will lead to an increase in heart rate, while increasing parasympathetic drive will lead to a decrease in heart rate.

Having briefly described these major constituents of the nervous system, it is appropriate to look at some of them more closely. The human brain weighs approximately 3 pounds. For purposes of description, it too can be divided into sections. One such division describes the brain in terms of three parts: the hindbrain, the midbrain, and the forebrain. Another uses the descriptors *brain stem, cerebellum,* and *cerebrum.* In both of these cases, the more basic functions are carried out by the first item in the list (i.e., hindbrain or brainstem) while the latter (i.e., forebrain or cerebrum) in each case is responsible for the most complex aspects of behavior and mental life. It is hard to make precise divisions, since all subdivisions are interconnected. For illustrative purposes, however, the brain can be thought of as three overlapping ovals; this representation is presented in Figure 2.2.

The three sections of the brain can be differentiated along an evolutionary time scale (see Ornstein & Sobel, 1990). Many millions of years ago, life forms were much more simple. Organisms consisted of a small number of cells, and they lived in water, which provided a constant environment as well as support for body weight (what little of it there was). As time progressed, life became more complex. Organisms grew larger and began to live on land (see Dawkins, 1989). Now, considerations such as keeping the body appropriately warm (thermoregulation), locomotion (involving musculoskeletal coordination), eating only every now and then (energy conservation and distribution), and dealing with a generally threatening environment (vision; perception of certain signals as indicating impending danger) became necessary. To deal with all these contingencies, many circuits of exquisite complexity evolved within the brain. Organizationally, these circuits are

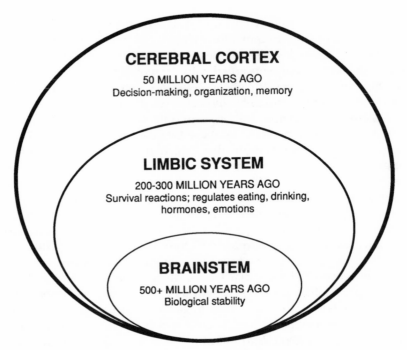

Figure 2.2. An evolutionary perspective of brain circuitry organization. While several descriptive classifications can be used for divisions of the brain, it is important to note that all subdivisions are interconnected by fiber tracts.

basically piled on top of each other, with the newest of them (those responsible for the so-called higher functions) being on top.

Blood pressure and heart rate are controlled by nuclei in the hindbrain, with the medulla being especially important, although the cerebellum and the hypothalamus may also be important as regards to heart rate (Andreassi, 1989). Another area of the brain of interest is the part of the forebrain called the *diencephalon*. This includes two structures of particular relevance to the topic of this volume, namely the thalamus and the hypothalamus. These structures are involved in emotion, and they are well connected to the sympathetic nervous system and the endocrine system. We shall see how these brain structures are important when considering the fight-or-flight response in Chapter 3.

Neurotransmitters and Receptors

A *neurotransmitter* is a naturally occurring (or *endogenous*) chemical messenger that passes a message from one neuron to the next by being released into the synaptic gap from the axon of the presynaptic neuron and then attaching itself to the receptor on the dendrite of the post-synaptic neuron. In addition to this natural process, two other possibilities can occur. Drugs can be introduced into the system; such drugs are *exogenous* compounds. There are two scenarios. The first concerns molecules called receptor *agonists*. These act very much in the same way as the neurotransmitter would. They are similar enough to the neurotransmitter to occupy the receptor site *and* similar enough for the dendrite to act as though the genuine, *endogenous* chemical neurotransmitter were present (i.e., as though the presynaptic cell had fired). The second scenario concerns the introduction of molecules called receptor *antagonists*. These molecules are similar enough to the genuine neurotransmitter to occupy the receptor sites but *not* similar enough for the dendrite to act as though the real neurotransmitter were present.

These *antagonists* thus occupy receptor sites without having a direct effect. However, they do have a very real indirect effect in that they prevent the neurotransmitter from being able to occupy the sites and thus prevent it from passing on its message. Thus, receptor antagonists are said to block the effect of the neurotransmitter. Such drugs are used in pharmacological studies called *blockade studies*. Blockade studies are used to investigate the mechanisms of a particular observed effect. If it is thought that a specific change in physiological activity is the result of a certain neurotransmitter, the receptor antagonist for that particular neurotransmitter can be introduced into the system. The antagonist will then occupy receptor sites and prevent the neurotransmitter from passing on its message. If the effect is no longer seen, this represents inferential evidence that the effect is indeed mediated by that particular neurotransmitter.

It should be noted here that, in the absence of externally administered drugs, neurons can pass on both excitatory and inhibitory messages when they fire. That is, the act of firing does not necessarily imply that the next neuron is likely to fire on receipt of this message; if an inhibitory message is passed on, the next neuron is *less* likely to fire. In this way, certain receptor antagonists can cause a particular effect to be *more* likely to happen. They do this by blocking the neurotransmitters carrying inhibitory messages. It should also be noted that some exogenous drugs exert their influence not by acting on the postsynaptic cell (at receptor sites) but by acting on the presynaptic cell (i.e., the cell that released the neurotransmitter in the first place). Normally, these neurotransmitters remain in the synaptic gap for only a short time; most are reabsorbed by the axon that secreted them. This process is called *reuptake*. However, drugs may block this reuptake process by occupying the sites on the axon at which reuptake occurs. This means that the neurotransmitter remains in the synaptic gap longer, influencing the postsynaptic cell for a longer period of time.

One particular class of receptors is of special interest here. The catecholamines *epinephrine* and *norepinephrine* initiate many physiological events by binding to specific target cell recognition sites, the *adrenergic receptors* (Mills & Dimsdale, 1988). We are presently interested in their influence on heart rate, myocardial contractility, vasoconstriction and vasodilation, and hence blood pressure. Two types of adrenergic receptors have been postulated (see Ahlquist, 1976a–c). These are known as *alpha* and *beta* adrenergic receptors, and they are often represented by the Greek letters α and β. Alpha-adrenergic receptors appears to be specific to the vasculature, and when stimulated, they lead to vasoconstriction. Beta-adrenergic receptors are found in the heart and in the vasculature. When stimulated, those in the heart lead to increased heart rate and contractile (myocardial) force, and those in the vasculature lead to vasodilation (Obrist, 1981).

The effects of sympathetic stimulation of the heart are thus straightforward: Sympathetic stimulation leads to a faster heart rate and greater contractile force. Epinephrine and norepinephrine both act as beta agonists on the heart. Both chemicals therefore induce increases in heart rate and myocardial contractile force. The effects of sympathetic stimulation of the vasculature, however, are more complex: It can result in both vasoconstrictive and vasodilatory effects, depending on which type of receptor is stimulated. Alpha-adrenergic excitation by the agonists norepinephrine and epinephrine leads to vasoconstriction. Beta-adrenergic stimulation of the vasculature by the agonist epinephrine leads to vasodilation. (For further discussions of adrenergic receptors, see Girdler *et al.*, 1992; Insel & Motulsky, 1987; Mills & Dimsdale, 1988, 1993; Robertson *et al.*, 1989; Sherwood & Hinderliter, 1993).

Higher Nervous Control of Cardiovascular Function

The autonomic nervous system plays prominent roles in many aspects of cardiovascular control (Rushmer, 1989). The parasympathetic nervous system, acting via the vagus nerve, acts on the heart to slow heart rate, but has little direct influence on the vasculature. The sympathetic nervous system acts to increase heart rate, and also exerts influence on the vasculature. As we shall see when considering the heart in the following section, parasympathetic influence is the dominant one under resting conditions. However, since the focus of the present volume is on cardiovascular activity and changes that occur during stress, it is appropriate now to consider the nervous system influences that operate under those circumstances.

During times of stress, external control of the heart can shift from the parasympathetic system to the sympathetic nervous system and the hormonal system. Thus, consideration of cardiovascular stress responses requires that we examine the necessary details of the system that secretes hormones. This is called the *endocrine system*, and it operates under the control of the central nervous system.

The Endocrine System

The endocrine system, like the nervous system, is a class of cells that can communicate with one another in ways that affect behavior (Bernstein *et al.*, 1991). This system, however, uses different methods to achieve this communication. Whereas the nervous system employs chemical neurotransmitters secreted into synaptic gaps, the endocrine cells group together into organs called *endocrine glands*. These glands secrete chemical messengers, called *hormones*, into the bloodstream, which carries the hormones to their target organs.

Hormones are chemicals similar to neurotransmitters; indeed, some chemicals act as both hormones and neurotransmitters. However, a major difference concerns how these substances are able to exert their influence. Neurotransmitters can only influence neurons they come into contact with, traveling over the very small gaps at synapses. In contrast, hormones can stimulate cells distant from their points of origin because they are secreted into the bloodstream, which then carries them throughout the body (Bernstein *et al.*, 1991). Cells that the hormones are able to stimulate have receptors for that particular hormone. Another major difference between neurotransmitters and hormones concerns the length of time for which they exert their influence. Neurotransmitters exert their influence for a brief period only. The release of neurotransmitters by axons is short lived, and reuptake or chemical decomposition of them normally takes place quickly. Consequently, they are only able to influence the receptors on adjacent dendrites for a brief time. In contrast, when hormones are released into the bloodstream they stay there for a much longer length of time, and they may affect many target organs.

Operation of Endocrine Glands

Some of the major glands of the endocrine system are the pituitary, hypothalamus, thyroid, parathyroid, pancreas, ovary, testis, and the adrenal glands. We shall pay attention to the adrenal glands (see next section), since they are involved in the fight-or-flight response discussed in the next chapter. However, the operation of each hormone is very similar in that secretion of each hormone is controlled by a feedback system.

The feedback loop usually has four elements: the brain, the pituitary gland, the endocrine organ, and the target organ, with the brain itself actually being one of the target organs. Bernstein et al. (1991) described the chain of events, with each element in the system using hormones to communicate with (i.e., influence or signal) the next element. The sequence is as follows:

In step one, the brain controls the pituitary gland by signaling the hypothalamus to release hormones that stimulate the receptors of the pituitary gland (the hypothalamus thus functions as an endocrine gland). In step two, the pituitary gland secretes one of its many different hormones. The secreted hormone then stimulates another endocrine gland to secrete its hormones. In the third step, these hormones act on the cells in the body. In the final step, the hormones themselves provide feedback to the brain and the pituitary gland. The feedback system thus regulates hormonal secretion. If the output of the final gland in this sequence does not reach a certain level, the hypothalamus and the pituitary continue to initiate secretion of more hormone. On the other hand, when the hormone level rises above a certain point, feedback signals cause the cessation of secretion. The brain (i.e., the central nervous system) therefore has ultimate control over the secretion of hormones.

The Adrenal Glands

The adrenal glands are located above the kidneys. They are involved in emotional arousal, including arousal under stress. Each adrenal gland has two parts. The outer part of each gland is called the *adrenal cortex*. The adrenal cortex releases the hormone *cortisol* when the central nervous system interprets a given situation as threatening, or stressful. Cortisol release is the result of activation of the brain-pituitary-endocrine gland connection mentioned above. Here, it is called the hypothalamic-pituitary-adrenal cortex axis.

When stimulated by the hypothalamus, the pituitary secretes adrenocorticotrophic hormone, which stimulates the adrenal cortex and controls its secretion of corticosteroids. One category of corticosteroids is the glucocorticoids, which help regulate glucose levels in the blood. Most of the glucocorticoid secretion in humans is cortisol (Gatchel *et al.*, 1989). Cortisol is very important in stress reactions. It has several effects on carbohydrate metabolism, increasing the body's access to energy stores of fats and carbohydrates, thus supporting arousal. Cortisol also inhibits inflammation of damaged body tissues (Gatchel *et al.*, 1989).

The inner part of each adrenal gland, the *adrenal medulla*, is innervated by the sympathetic nervous system. When the adrenal medulla is stimulated, it releases the catecholamines epinephrine (also called *adrenaline*) and norepinephrine (also called *noradrenaline*) into the bloodstream. However, contrary to fairly common belief, it is actually only epinephrine that acts on the cardiovascular system as a true hormone under normal circumstances (Folkow, 1982).[1] One of the many effects of circulating epinephrine is to increase the force with which the heart contracts, thereby influencing blood pressure. For a given heart rate, an increase in the contractile force of each beat will increase systolic pressure. In addition, epinephrine increases heart rate.

The overall effect of the hormones released by the adrenal glands during stress is to generate emergency energy in the body. Blood pressure is increased via increased heart rate and blood flow, the liver converts and releases some of its supply of stored sugar into the bloodstream, and the body's metabolism (the rate at which it uses

[1]Even though norepinephrine is indeed released from the adrenal medulla, it has limited, if any, hormonal action and almost certainly none on the walls of blood vessels. For further details, see the excellent review by Folkow (1982, p. 419). In its capacity as a sympathetic nervous system neurotransmitter, however, norepinephrine does indeed exert influence upon the vasculature.

energy) is considerably increased (Lahey, 1992). In conjunction with the actions of the sympathetic nervous system on the heart and blood vessels, this pattern of activation is known as the fight-or-flight syndrome.

The Cardiovascular System

The cardiovascular system's basic function is to provide oxygen and nutrients to sustain the living tissues contained within the body. However, to achieve that goal, which can be stated simply, the cardiovascular system has evolved to a phenomenal level of intricateness; the description provided in this chapter only begins to hint at the system's true sophistication.

Figure 2.3 presents a schematic diagram of the cardiovascular system. Also included is the respiratory system, since this system and the cardiovascular system interact. Blood is sent from the heart to the lungs to obtain oxygen. This oxygenated blood is channeled back to the heart and then pumped to the rest of the body to provide tissues with oxygen. Once these tissues have removed this oxygen, the deoxygenated blood is channeled back to the heart, where the process starts again. The pulmonary artery carries deoxygenated blood to the lungs, and the pulmonary vein carries oxygenated blood to the heart. This pulmonary circulation is thus the opposite of all other circulation, in which arteries carry oxygenated blood from the heart and veins carry deoxygenated blood back to the heart. The term *systemic vasculature* is used to refer to all vasculature except that in the pulmonary circulating subsystem. In this volume, considerations of the body's vasculature will focus entirely on the systemic vasculature.

The Heart

Structure

The human heart is a muscle that weighs about 300 g in the adult male and 250 g in the female. It contains four chambers: the right atrium and the right ventricle; and the left atrium and the left ventricle. In Figure 2.3, these are represented by RA, RV, LA, and LV, respectively. Blood returns from bodily tissues into the right atrium and then passes into the right ventricle, from where it is ejected into the pulmonary

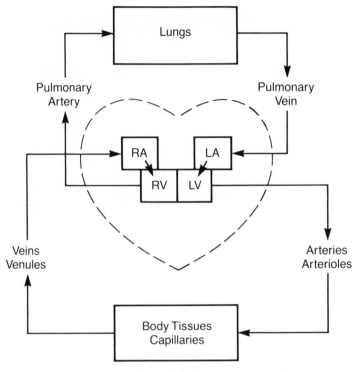

Figure 2.3. A schematic diagram of the cardiovascular system. Shown are both the pulmonary circulation (which takes blood from the heart to the lungs and back) and the systemic vasculature (all the vasculature except that in the pulmonary system). In this volume we shall focus on the heart and the systemic vasculature.

artery. Freshly oxygenated blood returns from the lungs to the left atrium, from where it passes into the left ventricle. Ejection into the aorta, and thus the body's arteries, occurs from this chamber. The motion of blood through the heart's chambers is governed by the opening and closing of the heart valves that connect the various heart chambers, and by the regular sequence of contraction and relaxation of the heart muscle (Gatchel *et al.*, 1989).

The phases of contraction and relaxation are the two constituents of the cardiac cycle. They are called *systole* and *diastole*, respectively. The cardiac cycle is commonly called the *heartbeat*. Heart rate, the number of cardiac cycles in a given time, is usually expressed in beats per minute (bpm). A normal heart will contract and relax (i.e., beat) approximately 70 times per minute for about 70 years or more, for a total of roughly two-and-a-half billion heartbeats. With each contraction, the powerful muscle fibers around the left ventricle eject blood into the aorta very forcefully.

Excitation of the Heart

The internal mechanisms for the regulation of heartbeats consist of several specialized fibers. Being a muscle, the heart requires an electrical stimulus to initiate its action. The normal heartbeat starts with the propagation of an electrical impulse in the sinoatrial node, the heart's natural pacemaker, which is located near the top of the right atrium. The regular electrical discharge from this node produces the usual rhythmic contraction of the entire heart. The impulse spreads through the atrial muscles, causing them to contract. This contraction is registered by the atrioventricular node, located at the bottom of the atrium, and conveyed via the Purkinje system to the ventricular muscles, causing ventricular systole. This series of contractions is preceded by a minute change in voltage (depolarization), which can be monitored at the body surface as the electrocardiogram, or ECG.

The ECG is probably the most commonly recognized bodily pattern of activity. In the late nineteenth century, it was realized that the electrical changes occurring during the heart's contraction could be detected by placing electrodes on the skin and connecting them to a galvanometer. These early recording practices have evolved via the pen-and-ink chart recorder to electrical monitors that display the signals (such as those seen in hospital use), and to computer systems that not only display the signals but also concurrently digitize them and store them for later re-creation and examination.

The ECG consists of three major components; these are the P-wave, the QRS complex, and the T-wave. These components, shown in Figure 2.4, are associated with atrial activity, excitation of the ventricles, and repolarization of the ventricles, respectively. Following contraction, the muscle relaxes to fill with blood again, and there is a refractory period during which time the muscle is unable to contract again. The length of the refractory period is determined by the rate of repolarization (Brener, 1967).

The sinoatrial node (the pacemaker), which is under the influence of both the sympathetic and the parasympathetic nervous systems, sets

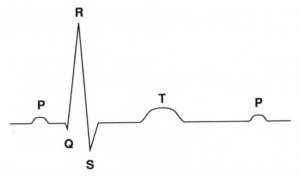

Figure 2.4. The electrocardiogram (ECG). Shown are the P-wave, the QRS complex, and the T-wave. While the skilled diagnostician can detect various abnormalities of cardiac function from examining the ECG, such considerations are beyond the scope of this volume. We shall focus on heart rate. To determine this, the number of R-waves are usually counted over a 1-minute interval, since the R-wave is the easiest landmark in the ECG for either the human eye or a computer system to detect.

a rate of 120 bpm at normal body temperature (Andreassi, 1989). However, the vagus nerve (part of the parasympathetic nervous system) inhibits the node, with the result that the actual resting heart rate is kept down to somewhere in the range of 70–80 bpm, with 72 bpm being an often-cited value. The vagus exerts its influence by releasing the neuro-transmitter *acetylcholine* at the nerve endings, which results in a slowing of the activity at the pacemaker, and also a slowing of the cardiac impulse passing into the ventricles (Guyton, 1977a). The sympathetic nervous system exerts its influence by releasing the neurotransmitter *norepinephrine* at the sympathetic nerve endings. This stimulation acts mainly at the pacemaker, increasing the rate of sinoatrial node discharge and accelerating atrio-ventricular conduction of impulses.

Under normal circumstances, then, when a healthy individual is resting, parasympathetic tone is predominant. If this parasympathetic influence is blocked by the administration of the appropriate drug (atropine), the heart speeds up considerably, demonstrating what is called a pronounced tachycardia or "high heart rate." (The equivalent term for slowing of the heart is bradycardia.) The fact that the parasym-pathetic tone is the dominant one under resting conditions can be shown by blocking the sympathetic innervation of the sinoatrial node (using propranolol); only a slight slowing of heart rate occurs (Berne &

Levy, 1986). Thus, removing parasympathetic (in this case, vagal) influence causes a big increase in heart rate, demonstrating that the vagus is exerting considerable control in keeping heart rate down; conversely, removing sympathetic influence results in only a small decrease in heart rate, showing that its normal excitatory influence under conditions of rest is only minimal.

Cardiac Output

The output of the heart, called cardiac output, is the amount of blood ejected in a given unit of time. As with heart rate, cardiac output is usually represented in intervals of a minute. Cardiac output is determined by heart rate and by stroke volume, which is the amount of blood ejected per beat. Stroke volume is usually measured in milliliters (ml) per beat, and cardiac output in liters per minute (lpm). The relationship among heart rate, stroke volume, and cardiac output can be expressed mathematically as:

$$\text{Cardiac output} = \text{heart rate} \times \text{stroke volume}$$

At rest, cardiac output is about 5 to 6 lpm, but there is a reserve of as much as 25 lpm (Wilson *et al.*, 1989).

The Vasculature

Structure

The vasculature consists of arteries, arterioles, capillaries, venules, and veins. Arteries branching out from the aorta carry blood to all parts of the body. Arteries are made up of layers of smooth muscle fibers and elastic membrane tissue, a combination that allows them to stretch when blood is forced through them at high pressure and then easily return to normal when pressure is relaxed (Andreassi, 1989). Arterioles carry blood into capillary beds, where exchange of nutrients and waste products occurs in bodily tissues. Capillaries are only about 0.017 mm in diameter, and they bring circulating blood to within about 0.1 mm from most cells in the body (Rushmer, 1989). The capillary networks, which would have a combined length of about 60,000 miles, present an enormous surface area to body tissues so that only 5 liters of blood can serve the entire body of a person weighing 70 kilograms (kg), or 154 pounds (Rushmer, 1989). Blood leaves the capillary beds via small venules, which become the veins that carry the blood back to the heart.

Innervation of Blood Vessels

All blood vessels (with the exception of the capillaries) are innervated by the sympathetic nervous system only; the parasympathetic system exerts no direct control over the peripheral blood vessels (Gardner, 1975; Guyton, 1977a). The sympathetic nervous system is responsible here for both the increase and decrease in diameter of the blood vessels (vasodilation and vasoconstriction, respectively).

The vasomotor center of the medulla maintains sympathetic vasoconstrictor tone; the vasoconstrictor fibers of the sympathetic nervous system innervate the arteries, arterioles, and veins (Berne & Levy, 1986). Normal sympathetic tone keeps almost all of the blood vessels of the body constricted to about half of their maximum diameter (Andreassi, 1989). Increases in sympathetic activation of alpha-adrenergic receptors in the cardiovascular system lead to further constriction, whereas increasing activation of beta-adrenergic receptors leads to a decrease in vasoconstriction (i.e., vasodilation). The degree of vasoconstriction is important because it is directly related to the resistance the vasculature presents to the flow of blood through it. The combined resistance of the systemic vasculature to blood flow is called *total peripheral resistance*. The greater the degree of vasoconstriction, the greater the resistance. Conversely, as vasodilation increases, the resistance of the vasculature decreases. The resistance of the vasculature is important because it directly affects blood pressure. Therefore, vasoconstriction and vasodilation are also directly related to blood pressure.

Arterial Blood Pressure

There is continuous pressure in the arteries to provide the driving force necessary to propel blood through the capillaries and back to the heart through the venous system (Rushmer, 1989). The actual level of pressure normally fluctuates between about 120 millimeters of mercury (mmHg) and 80 mmHg, with this fluctuation occurring during each cardiac cycle. The unit of measurement of blood pressure (i.e., millimeters of mercury) is used because the pressure, if channeled to the bottom of a column of mercury, would cause the mercury to rise a certain number of millimeters in height. The first invasive methods of measuring blood pressure employed such a mercury column, and the height of the mercury varied a given number of millimeters throughout each cardiac cycle. A modified, noninvasive version of this procedure is used each time a person's blood pressure is taken in the doctor's office using a mercury sphygmomanometer.

The higher level of blood pressure in the arteries occurs upon ejection of blood into the arterial tree. This occurs during the phase of the cardiac cycle called *systole*. This higher level of pressure is termed *systolic blood pressure* (SBP). The lower level of pressure occurs between bouts of ejection, during *diastole*. This pressure is called *diastolic blood pressure* (DBP). Systolic pressure can be thought of as being an indicator of the maximum pressure with which blood is ejected from the heart during the peak contraction during systole, while diastolic pressure can be regarded as a representation of the steady pressure within the vasculature between beats. For young adult males, the previously cited values of 120 mmHg and 80 mmHg are often considered average levels for systolic and diastolic pressure, respectively. Pressures for females tend to be somewhat lower, while pressures typically increase in both genders with age.

Two other blood pressure parameters of interest are pulse pressure and mean arterial pressure. *Pulse pressure* is the difference between systolic and diastolic pressure. The values of 120 mmHg and 80 mmHg, respectively, would therefore give a pulse pressure of 40 mmHg. *Mean arterial pressure* (MAP) is a way of expressing a representative pressure over the entire cardiac cycle. Mean arterial pressure is calculated as diastolic blood pressure plus one-third pulse pressure; that is,

$$MAP = DBP + 1/3 \, (SBP - DBP)$$

It is worth noting here that although the word "mean" appears in the term "mean arterial pressure," this value is *not* the arithmetic mean of systolic and diastolic pressure. The values of 120 mmHg and 80 mmHg (for systolic and diastolic pressure, respectively) yield a mean arterial pressure of 93.3 mmHg.

Mean arterial pressure is ultimately determined by a cardiac factor and a vascular factor—namely cardiac output (CO) and total peripheral resistance of the systemic vasculature (TPR). The relationship between these two hemodynamic parameters and blood pressure is expressed in the following equation:

$$\text{Mean arterial blood pressure} =$$
$$\text{Cardiac output} \times \text{Total peripheral resistance}$$

Expressed using the usual abbreviations, this equation is:

$$MAP = CO \times TPR$$

Arterial blood pressure can therefore be thought of as representing a manifestation of the interaction between the heart and the vasculature (Obrist, 1981). If either cardiac output or peripheral resistance increases while the other remains constant, an increase in pressure will occur. A given change in blood pressure can therefore be the result of a change in cardiac output or a change in peripheral resistance (or a combination of changes in both). Encapsulated within this simple relationship is the basis for much of the current excitement within cardiovascular behavioral medicine concerning the assessment of the hemodynamic bases of blood pressure changes in different individuals and situations. This will be discussed in the next chapter.

Renal Influences on Cardiovascular Function

Although the kidneys are not part of the cardiovascular system, they can have a profound influence on cardiovascular functioning (Obrist, 1981). Their primary role is the maintenance of body fluid volume and chemical (electrolyte) balance. Fluid and salt balances are kept within very narrow limits. To do this, the kidneys excrete urine. The composition of the urine depends on the total amount of body fluids and their chemical composition. For example, if more water or sodium is ingested than is needed, the kidneys will excrete the surplus.

More than half of the body weight of humans is due to water. An average person weighing 70 kg contains about 40 liters of water (Rushmer, 1989). About 60% of this water is intracellular fluid (located within body cells). Of the body's extracellular fluid, about 5 liters comprise the total blood volume. It is important that total blood volume is kept constant since this too is a determinant of blood pressure. If blood volume increases, blood pressure increases because of a greater amount of fluid within a fixed system. The kidneys respond to this increased pressure by excreting fluid at a higher rate, returning fluid volume and hence blood pressure to normal. It is also true that the kidneys will reduce their excretion if blood volume falls below the level necessary for the desired blood pressure.

While the main focus of this book is short-term regulation of blood pressure, and also possible long-term consequences of such regulation, it should be acknowledged here that some authorities emphasize the role of the renal system in the long-term regulation of blood pressure. Dr. Arthur Guyton has argued that chronic hypertension probably never occurs without abnormal function of the renal system, and that fluid excretion by the kidneys plays the overriding role in determining the long-term level to which blood pressure is regulated (Guyton, 1989).

Renal function involves the steady filtering of total body water through rapid recycling of plasma fluid (Falkner, 1989). This is accomplished by three aspects of kidney activity: (1) glomerular filtration, (2) tubular reabsorption, and (3) tubular secretion. What Dr. Guyton and colleagues have proposed is that the kidneys operate most efficiently at a set pressure level in terms of their ability to excrete sodium and water from the body (Hollandsworth, 1986). This pressure level is called the *set point*. If this set point should be raised, the kidneys will retain fluid until blood volume is sufficient to raise blood pressure to this new level; excretion rates will then maintain this new set point. Sympathetic activity can affect the set point in various ways: These include a direct neural effect on sodium reabsorption, an effect on renal hemodynamics that modifies the physical forces involved in sodium reabsorption, and an effect on the secretion of hormones influencing sodium reabsorption (Hollandsworth, 1986).

Although renal regulation of blood pressure is much slower than regulation by the autonomic nervous system, long-term renal determination of blood pressure may be very important, and the reader is referred to Falkner (1989), Guyton (1989), and Pitts (1974) for more detailed overviews.

Respiratory Influences on Cardiovascular Function

The respiratory system and the cardiovascular system interact when blood is sent to the lungs in order to obtain the oxygen it then distributes to body tissues. In addition to this process of blood oxygenation, the respiratory system also influences cardiac functioning. Two types of respiratory-cardiac coordination are respiratory sinus arrhythmia and hyperventilation-induced cardiac changes (Grossman & Wientjes, 1985).

Respiratory sinus arrhythmia is the name given to the cyclic fluctuations in heart rate that occur during respiration. Generally, heart rate increases during inspiration and decreases during expiration. The interbeat interval is the time, usually measured in milliseconds, between two consecutive heartbeats. The faster the heart beats, the shorter the interbeat interval. During inspiration, then, the interbeat interval becomes smaller, and during expiration it becomes greater.

Respiratory sinus arrhythmia amplitude is defined as the difference between the minimum and maximum interbeat intervals. In practice, the assessment of respiratory sinus arrhythmia requires sophisticated statistical procedures, since other influences are operating upon heart rate simultaneously. However, it is being increasingly used in psychophysiological studies as an index of vagal tone. As Berntson, Cacioppo, and Quigley (1993) commented in a recent comprehensive review of respiratory sinus arrhythmia, it may be among the most selective noninvasive indices of parasympathetic control of cardiac functions.

The role of sympathetic activation in stress responses is widely acknowledged and well documented, and this text concentrates on such activation. However, the possible involvement of the parasympathetic nervous system in stress response has to date received considerably less experimental investigation. Although there have been some investigations of parasympathetic influence using pharmacological blockade, there have been few psychophysiological studies reported that examined cardiac parasympathetic influences in relation to hypertension under nonpharmacological conditions (Grossman *et al.*, 1992). The availability of a noninvasive index of vagal tone, such as respiratory sinus arrhythmia, is therefore important.

Because the heart is dually innervated by the sympathetic and parasympathetic nervous systems, the parasympathetic system provides mechanisms that could attenuate sympathetically mediated heart rate responses to stress, and it might have more general antagonistic actions on stress reactivity (Lane *et al.*, 1992). That is, individuals who have higher levels of parasympathetic tone might, through such mechanisms, be less reactive when stressors elicit sympathetically mediated responses (Lane *et al.*, 1992).

Although this volume concentrates on sympathetic activation and sympathetically mediated responses during psychological stress, it should be noted here that it will be important to monitor the future study of parasympathetic influence (and the sympathetic/parasympathetic balance of influence; see Berntson *et al.*, 1991) during stress responses, and to evaluate its predictive powers in terms of cardiovascular stress reactivity and the risk for cardiovascular disease (Lane *et al.*, 1992). (See also Friedman *et al.*, 1993; Grossman *et al.*, 1991; Miller, 1993; and Porges, 1985, 1986.)

Integration of Nervous, Endocrine, and Cardiovascular Systems

This chapter has provided a brief and very selective introduction to these three bodily systems. This information will provide a basis for the discussions of cardiovascular responses during psychological stressors in later chapters. Accordingly, the links among the three systems have been emphasized since, in the situations we shall examine, they operate in an integrated manner.

Figure 2.5 is a diagrammatic representation of this integration. The figure contains six units. Beginning at the top, the first unit represents the starting point of the entire process that we are interested in (i.e., cardiovascular response to stress). The first step in this process is the perception of a situation as stressful, and the system responsible for such perception is of course the nervous system. If cognitive appraisal—the process of situational analysis and assessment—defines a situation as challenging or threatening, a whole series of events occurs. We do not have to exert voluntary control to gear up our systems; the autonomic nervous system and the endocrine system are activated by the central nervous system.

The second unit in Figure 2.5 looks at some of the modifying influences in the subsequent chain of physiological outcomes; many of the items listed here will be discussed in later chapters. The third unit contains the communication network. Involved here are the nervous system and the endocrine system. Receptors are also mentioned. These are receiving increasing attention. An alteration in the sensitivity of these, or in the number of them (density), can alter the chemical effects of a certain amount of neurotransmitter; for example, a stronger message will be forwarded by more sensitive receptors (see Mills & Dimsdale [1988] for a review). The fourth unit in Figure 2.5 lists the cardiovascular system.

The fifth and sixth units represent the renal volume-pressure

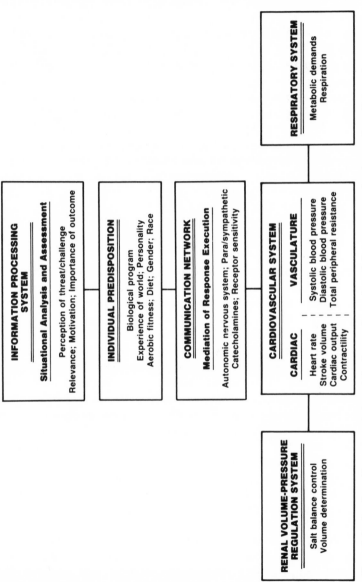

Figure 2.5. A schematic representation of the integrative action of the nervous, endocrine, and cardiovascular systems. Although the figure contains six units for the purposes of illustration, they are all interrelated. The figure represents a process whose very nature is integrative and interactive.

regulation system and the respiratory system, respectively. Although we shall not focus on these two systems in this text, renal and cardio-respiratory influences are important topics (see Allen *et al.*, 1986; Grossman, 1983; Guyton, 1989; these references are also listed at the end of this chapter).

Many different physiological systems operate in a highly integrated manner to produce the cardiovascular adjustments that are the focus of this book. In one sense, Figure 2.5 imposes artificial constraints and designations upon a process whose very nature is integrative and interactive. However, it does provide a concise representation of the many psychological and physiological processes that culminate in the seemingly simple occurrence of cardiovascular responses during a stressful situation.

Summary

The interaction of the nervous and cardiovascular systems is the focus of this text. During nonstressful periods, cardiovascular activity is matched to concurrent metabolic needs. When a situation is perceived as threatening or stressful, however, the central nervous system takes over. It exerts its influence on the cardiovascular system via the endocrine system and also by overriding normal autonomic functioning and increasing sympathetic nervous system outflow to the heart and sites of peripheral resistance in the peripheral vasculature (Rushmer, 1989). The pituitary gland causes the adrenal glands to secrete cortisol into the bloodstream. Epinephrine is also released from the adrenal glands as a hormone, but its release is governed directly by the sympathetic nervous system. Norepinephrine is released as a neurotransmitter during sympathetic activation of both the heart and the vasculature. Both catecholamines (epinephrine and norepinephrine) stimulate the cardiovascular system to help the body prepare to deal with the perceived imminent threat. Norepinephrine acts on the constrictor muscles of the systemic vasculature to stimulate further vasoconstriction. Norepinephrine and epinephrine increase heart rate and the contractile force with which the heart ejects blood. All of these influences act to increase blood pressure.

One of the major goals in the discipline of behavioral medicine is to address some of the overriding influences of the higher levels of the nervous system on organ function in health and disease (Rushmer,

1989). In the present volume, we are concerned with central nervous system control of cardiovascular function during stress. Stress can lead to considerable alteration of cardiovascular activity, and it is these responses that are the focus of cardiovascular reactivity research.

Further Reading

1. Allen, M.T., Sherwood, A., & Obrist, P.A. (1986). Interactions of respiratory and cardiovascular adjustments to behavioral stressors. *Psychophysiology, 23,* 532–541.
2. Asterita, M.F. (1985). *The physiology of stress—with special reference to the neuroendocrine system.* New York: Human Sciences Press.
3. Berne, R.M., & Levy, M.N. (1986). *Cardiovascular physiology* (5th ed.). St. Louis: Mosby.
4. Falkner, B. (1989). Measurement of volume regulation: Renal function. In N. Schneiderman, S.M. Weiss, & P.G. Kaufmann (Eds.), *Handbook of research methods in cardiovascular behavioral medicine* (pp. 117–129). New York: Plenum.
5. Grossman, P. (1983). Respiration, stress, and cardiovascular function. *Psychophysiology, 20,* 284–300.
6. Guyton, A.C. (1989). Dominant role of the kidneys and accessory role of whole-body autoregulation in the pathogenesis of hypertension. *American Journal of Hypertension, 2,* 575–585.
7. Mills, P.J., & Dimsdale, J.E. (1992). Sympathetic nervous system responses to psychosocial stressors. In J.R. Turner, A. Sherwood, & K.C. Light (Eds.), *Individual differences in cardiovascular response to stress* (pp. 33–49). New York: Plenum.
8. Rushmer, R.F. (1989). Structure and function of the cardiovascular system. In N. Schneiderman, S.M. Weiss, & P.G. Kaufmann (Eds.). *Handbook of research methods in cardiovascular behavioral medicine* (pp. 5–22). New York: Plenum.
9. Selye, H. (1976). *The stress of life* (rev. ed.). New York: McGraw-Hill.
10. Ziegler, M.G. (1989). Catecholamine measurement in behavioral research. In N. Schneiderman, S.M. Weiss, & P.G. Kaufmann (Eds.). *Handbook of research methods in cardiovascular behavioral medicine* (pp. 167–183). New York: Plenum.

CHAPTER 3

Modeling Stress and Assessing Reactivity in the Laboratory

Stress is now a fashionable public concern. However, the concept has been of interest to the medical profession for centuries (Gatchel *et al.*, 1989). At the beginning of the twentieth century, the work of Cannon (1927, 1929, 1935) formalized the notion of stress. Cannon was among the first to use the term *stress* in a nonengineering context (Carroll, 1992); the terms *stress* and *strain* have long been used in the physical sciences. Though a physiologist by training, Cannon was aware of psychological and emotional influences, stating that emotional stress could cause considerable physiological alterations and viewing stress as a potential cause of medical problems.

The scientific study of stress received an additional boost from the work of Selye (1956, 1976), whose work focused more on physiological than psychological aspects. Selye proposed that any kind of stressor leads to the same pattern of physiological activation, called the *general adaptation syndrome*. This syndrome has three stages: alarm, resistance, and exhaustion. Once the initial impact of the stressor has been absorbed, the body settles down to resist the long-term effects of the stressor if it persists. Eventually, however, the body becomes exhausted by this process, and pathophysiology is a likely consequence. Although Selye's work has quite rightly been influential, it is now generally acknowledged that, at least in humans, physiological stress responses do not adhere to this rigid model. Specific responses can vary from person to person. This model also pays relatively little attention to the natures of differing psychological and emotional stressors.

In contrast, Lazarus and colleagues (Lazarus, 1966; Lazarus & Folkman, 1984) have concentrated on the psychological dimension of the stress concept, although they certainly do not ignore the physiological responses. A basic premise of their work is that an individual has to perceive or interpret a situation as stressful in order for there to be a stress response. Psychological or cognitive appraisal therefore plays a considerable role in Lazarus and colleagues' theories.

One particular study (Lazarus *et al.*, 1965) provided elegant support for this perspective. Subjects in this study viewed a particularly unpleasant film depicting workers being maimed or killed by accidents occurring in a woodshop. The subjects were split into three groups prior to the study; two groups received instructions on how to appraise the contents of the film while viewing it. The "denial" group was told that actors were used to stage the accidents, and that no real injuries occurred. The "intellectualization" group was told to regard the film's content as useful information that could be employed in safety-awareness campaigns. Both of these groups displayed less alteration in heart rate while subsequently watching the film than did the group of subjects who received no prior instructions on how to appraise the film's contents.

It is clear from these considerations that when examining "stress" we must pay attention to both external and internal events. Looking only at the environment (environmental events are called *stressors*) or only at the effects (both biological and psychological) does not provide a complete picture. Thus, stress can be regarded as the process by which environmental events threaten or challenge an organism's well-being and by which that organism responds to this threat. It involves environmental and psychological events, interpretations of them, and behavioral and physiological responses (Gatchel *et al.*, 1989). As Lazarus and Launier (1978) observed, stress is a transaction between people and the environment.

Modeling Stress in the Laboratory

The work of Lazarus and colleagues has a clear implication for contemporary stress research. To study physiological responses to stress, we must create a situation that people appraise as stressful. A key question in cardiovascular reactivity research is: Can we create stressful situations in the experimental laboratory that will elicit the cardiovascular responses we wish to study? While it is true that ultimately, as behavioral scientists, we must study stress responses in their normal setting of contemporary everyday life (a topic discussed in Chapter 9), studying them in the cardiovascular psychophysiological laboratory, if possible, should prove extremely helpful. The laboratory provides a setting in which strict environmental control can be exerted, and this is extremely helpful in the early stages of creating and examining different theories.

The purpose of real-life fight-or-flight responses is to prepare the organism for immediate physical action—that is, to fight or to flee. Increased cardiovascular activity and the release of cortisol facilitate the additional nutritional supply needed for such exertion and the preparation to minimize any damage sustained to the body. The evolutionary significance of such preparation is clear. As Folkow and Neil (1971, p. 348) commented, "Beyond doubt, this cardiovascular-hormonal anticipatory adjustment is of the utmost importance for survival in the animal kingdom." However, in highly developed social contexts, the pattern of hazards is different from that faced by the hunter-gatherer. Although life in some sections of modern society is extremely perilous, contemporary challenges are often symbolic, not involving immediate physical threat or demanding mobilization for vigorous counteraction. Nevertheless, it seems that these challenges provoke much the same pattern of preparatory adjustments seen in the case of physical threat. The neurohormonal (neurohumoral) complex that drives the fight-or-flight reaction can therefore be elicited not only by potentially life-threatening situations, but also "by those which imply 'stimulating' or even amusing challenges for the individual" (Folkow & Neil, 1971, p. 569).

This observation has two implications. First, it means that moderate levels of arousal are elicited repeatedly during everyday life, and that neurohormonal links mobilize the cardiovascular system repeatedly. Second, it means that this response can be studied in the laboratory as long as the experimental tasks employed do indeed provide a stimulating challenge for the individual.

Several psychologically challenging stressors have been developed for use in laboratory studies. These stressors are deliberately constructed so that the physical component is very small, and quite often consists of moving one finger every few seconds to depress a response key. For present purposes, psychological stressors can be operationally defined by two criteria. They are those that (1) demand continuous mental effort and active engagement in the task in order to achieve reasonable task completion, and that (2) require minimal physical exertion. Using these criteria, the following four examples can clearly be classified as psychological stressors.

Reaction Time Tasks

The simplest form of the reaction time task is one where the subject sits quietly with one finger poised over a button or key. As soon as a stimulus (usually a light or a sound) is detected, the subject has to depress the key. The time from stimulus onset to the subject's reaction is measured electronically; this value is the reaction time for that trial. This basic form of the task, however, can be altered in several ways. For example, Obrist *et al.* (1974) employed the reaction time task in an avoidance paradigm. Subjects in this study were threatened with an electric shock (delivered via electrodes attached to their calf muscle) if their performance did not reach a criterion level. Because subjects had no way of knowing whether performance on any specific trial was adequate, an element of uncertainty was introduced (uncertainty is an underlying common element in many tasks that elicit large-magnitude cardiovascular responses in certain individuals).

Because threatening to give electrical shocks is not particularly pleasant (even if it is effective in producing heart rate increases), other versions of the simple reaction time task have been developed. One version involves offering a monetary incentive for good performance on each trial, and another involves direct head-to-head competition; these versions are called *appetitive* and *competitive* paradigms, respectively (see Light, 1981).

Mental Arithmetic

Mental arithmetic tasks have a long and venerable history in studies of physiological responsivity (e.g., Brod *et al.*, 1959). One form of this task is the serial subtraction task. Here, subjects are given a number (e.g., 1754) and asked to subtract 17 from this number, and then 17 from the resulting number, and so forth, saying each successive answer out loud. Subjects are usually encouraged during pretask instructions to be as fast and as accurate as possible in their responses. Modern versions of this task will sometimes incorporate incentives; bonus awards of 10 cents per correct answer during a 3-minute task period may be offered. Here, the subject may be stopped each time he or she gives a wrong answer and asked to start again from the last previously given correct answer. Another type of math task provides subjects with a series of problems such as "137 − 49" and allows a brief 1- or 2-second window after each problem during which the subject may respond. Incentives may again be offered to encourage continued engagement in the task.

Mental arithmetic tasks such as the two described above have the advantage of being ideally suited to standardized presentation, but they do have one drawback. Before considering the drawback, what do we mean by standardized presentation? Simply this: In psychophysiological experiments, as in any other experimental psychological study, each subject should be given exactly the same task in exactly the same manner. Giving subjects precisely the same questions in the same sequence and at precisely the same temporal intervals, which the second previous example does, is a very good example of standardized task presentation. Yet, ironically, this very standardization can be problematic if the subject sample in a particular study is drawn from a population whose members differ widely in the relevant skill, namely mathematical ability. One way around this problem is to use an interactive task such as MATH (see Turner *et al.*, 1986b, 1987b). MATH is an interactive program that presents subjects with problems of a level of difficulty continuously determined by the accuracy of subjects' previous responses. Accurate responses lead to harder problems being presented, whereas incorrect answers lead to easier problems.

This interactive math task can be thought of as incorporating standardized flexibility. While the same task is used for everyone, the task is inherently flexible; one intrinsic permutation of possible problems will be appropriate for every member of a very heterogeneous subject population, and every member will thus be equally challenged. In this manner, the task is able to stimulate the cardiovascular systems of all individuals sufficiently and equally such that those who are predisposed to show increases do so, and those who are not predisposed do not. It is this activation of a threshold-based delineation between high reactors (those showing sizable reactivity) and low reactors that, from many points of view, is the most important characteristic of any task used in this research field.

Other scientists have also developed flexible tasks with the aim of extending research beyond the behavioral medicine laboratory and into the community. One aim in this research area is to develop a battery of tasks that can be easily administered to large-scale subject samples. Standardized tasks and the advent of portable computer systems help enormously in this goal. One research group has proposed a highly standardized battery of computer-based cognitive tasks with this aim in mind (Kamarck *et al.*, 1992). Such broad-based reactivity assessment will be examined in more detail in Chapter 10.

Video Games

Another category from which several tasks have been chosen is that of video games. Early studies employing games such as video tennis and handball showed them to have considerable cardiovascular impact. Glass *et al.* (1980) employed a two-person video game called "Super Pong." In this game, which is similar to tennis or hockey, each player attempts to score a goal with an electronic "ball." An average heart rate increase of 16.3 bpm was found. Dembroski *et al.* (1981) used a game similar to handball or squash, in which the subject is required to keep the "ball" in play by manipulating a desk-mounted control lever. Mean heart rate increase was 16.9 bpm. Turner *et al.* (1983) employed a "Space Invaders" video game (see also Turner, 1989). This particular video game embodied elements of uncertainty, novelty, and avoidance (all of which are important in generating continued task engagement on the part of the subject), although the consequences of nonavoidance in this case are nonaversive; unlike the reaction time task discussed earlier, the consequence of poor performance on this video game task is symbolically failing to save the world from extraterrestrial invaders rather than receiving a painful shock to the leg.

Finally, some of these video games contain the element of standardized flexibility discussed in the previous section. In the "Space Invaders" video game, the subject has command of a spaceship with which to attempt to destroy the ever-encroaching enemy craft. The subject's task is to do so before their constant barrage of missiles destroys his or her own spaceship, thus leaving Earth defenseless. However, the pace of the game speeds up as it progresses; as an increasing percentage of the enemy craft is destroyed, their missiles fall more quickly. Thus, the higher the level of the subject's skill the more difficult the game becomes. In this manner, each subject is faced with an appropriate level of task difficulty.

Speech Tasks

Recent studies employing psychophysiological techniques in the context of behavioral medicine have increasingly adopted speech tasks as one of their laboratory stressors. One version of the speech task requires subjects to read a passage during a preparatory period (perhaps 3 minutes) and then to present the information contained within the article as clearly and concisely as possible (e.g., see Girdler *et al.*, 1990). Subjects may be informed that their talk during the presentation period will be recorded and evaluated later for content, clarity, and interest.

A second version of this task, and one that is more commonly used, requires subjects to construct a story or scenario around the interpersonal interactions that might take place during a hypothetical stressful situation (see Saab *et al.*, 1989). One scenario is being denied permission to board an aircraft to fly to a very important meeting some considerable distance away (Girdler *et al.*, 1990). Another is being arrested and falsely accused of shoplifting. This second version of the speech task again displays the advantage of standardized flexibility. Each subject is given the same task under the same testing conditions, yet every subject brings to bear his or her own levels of verbal ability and imagination.

A Different Type of Stressor: The Cold Pressor

Finally, it is appropriate to describe another task that has long been used in research on hypertension (see Fredrikson & Matthews, 1990). The cold pressor task simply involves putting one's hand or foot into a bucket of ice water, or, more recently, having a bag of ice water placed on one's forehead (see Durel *et al.*, 1993; Peckerman *et al.*, 1991; Saab *et al.*, 1993; see also Lovallo, 1975).

While this task is quite clearly different from the four tasks just described, the precise classification of the cold pressor has proved problematic (Pickering & Gerin, 1990). It is not a psychological stressor, since it does not meet the first of our criteria: It does not require continuous mental effort and active engagement in the task in order to achieve reasonable task completion. All one has to do is to sit still and have ice water applied to one's body! The cold pressor has, therefore, been called a *passive* stressor, as opposed to an *active* stressor.

Obrist (1976) discussed the "activity-passivity dimension," conceptualizing the difference between psychologically engaging tasks (such as reaction time tasks) and tasks such as the cold pressor as requiring active and passive coping, respectively. The cold pressor has also been called a *physical* stressor, as opposed to a *psychological* stressor, thus placing it in a category with exercise tasks, for example. However, neither the active/passive nor psychological/physical dichotomies may capture the full complexity of the difference between the cold pressor and other tasks. It is possible that, while the nature of the cold pressor task itself requires no ongoing mental engagement for successful completion, some individuals may use various types of mental strategies in an attempt to avoid focusing on the pain caused by the task.

In contrast to these classification problems, however, a more recent way of looking at different stressors presents a clearer picture. We shall see later in the chapter that a system of task categorization that pays attention to the hemodynamic patterns of response elicited by different tasks allows the cold pressor to be placed unambiguously into a certain category within that system.

Assessment of Laboratory Reactivity

Once we have chosen laboratory tasks that will elicit changes in cardiovascular activity, we need to pay attention to two further considerations in order to study this reactivity. First, we have to equip the laboratory with suitable measurement devices that will allow us to measure physiological activity during various experimental periods of time.[1] Second, we have to decide exactly how reactivity is to be defined. In Chapter 1, we defined reactivity in terms of its computation as a change score, representing the change in physiological activity between a resting baseline period and a task period. While this computational definition is accurate, a more rigorous definition is also provided in this chapter.

Physiological Measures

Although a considerable array of measures can be employed in modern cardiovascular psychophysiological strategies, we shall focus on those most commonly used in behavioral medicine paradigms. Considered below, therefore, is the measurement of heart rate, blood pressure, cardiac output, and total peripheral resistance. For descrip-

---

[1]The word "measure" may not be the most precise here, but it is used judiciously to convey the appropriate sentiment. Leaving aside the philosophical considerations concerning the feasibility of any precise measurement, it is conceded that words such as "assess" or "derive" may be more suitable. In some cases, so too might "estimate," as long as it is realized that the estimates are made with a high degree of confidence.

tive purposes, these are presented individually, but it is worth reiterating that experimental attention in a given study often focuses on several, if not all, of these parameters.

Heart Rate

Heart rate is probably the most frequently measured variable in cardiovascular psychophysiology. One of the reasons for this is that it can be measured easily and accurately. The simplest way is to count pulses at the wrist while using a stopwatch. In the psychophysiology laboratory, however, it is more common to instrument subjects with electrodes and monitor their electrocardiograms. To obtain a statement of heart rate, R-waves can be counted by hand if the ECG is recorded on a pen-and-ink polygraph chart, or by a computer if the signal is monitored electronically.

Blood Pressure

The two main categories of blood pressure measurement techniques are *direct* and *indirect*. The true measurement of blood pressure can only be achieved by the direct method, which involves placing a sensing device into an artery (Andreassi, 1989). However, as you can imagine, direct measurement of intra-arterial blood pressure would be problematic in the psychophysiological laboratory. Apart from the subject's discomfort, and distraction from the experimental tasks, there is also the slight risk of medical complications. Therefore, indirect blood pressure measurement techniques are usually employed.

The most common indirect technique involves the use of a blood pressure cuff, a sphygmomanometer, and a stethoscope. The cuff is placed around the upper portion of the arm and is then inflated to a fairly high pressure—for example, 180 mmHg. The idea is to inflate the cuff sufficiently so that the artery is collapsed; that is, no blood is able to flow because the pressure in the cuff is greater than the pressure propelling the blood. If this is achieved (as it usually will be at 180 mmHg), the stethoscope, which has been placed over the brachial artery, detects no noise because there is no blood flow.

The cuff pressure is then gradually reduced, which means the pressure applied to the arm, and hence the artery, is reduced. Eventually, a pressure is reached when blood starts to spurt through the artery with each heart beat. The sounds made by the passing blood, called

Korotkoff sounds after the method's founder, are detected via the stethoscope. The person performing the blood pressure measurement notes the pressure registered on the sphygmomanometer when the first sound is heard. This value is designated the *systolic blood pressure*. With further cuff pressure reduction, blood flows more and more easily until the flow becomes unimpeded and hence continuous. At this point, Korotkoff sounds are no longer heard; the pressure at which they disappear is designated the *diastolic blood pressure*. (See Steptoe, 1980, for a more detailed discussion of blood pressure.)

Cardiac Output

The noninvasive measurement of cardiac output in the psychophysiology laboratory has been facilitated by the technique of *impedance cardiography* (see Hurwitz *et al.*, 1993; Hurwitz *et al.*, 1990; Miller & Horvath, 1978; Nagel *et al.*, 1989; Sherwood, 1993; Sherwood *et al.*, 1990a; Wilson *et al.*, 1989).

Four band electrodes, or an array of spot electrodes (see Sherwood *et al.*, 1992b), are typically placed around the subject, two above and two below the level of the aorta. A very small, very high frequency alternating electrical current (which is completely harmless to biological tissues) is introduced into the thorax via the two outer electrodes, while the two inner electrodes are used to measure surface potential.

Surface potential is directly proportional to the resistance to the flow of the current being passed. Resistance associated with alternating current is known as *impedance*. The main contributor to the changes in impedance seen during each cardiac cycle is the amount of blood flowing into the aorta (and therefore being ejected by the heart into the arterial tree). Since blood is a good conductor, greater decreases in impedance are associated with greater amounts of blood. This relationship can be used to determine stroke volume. Once a representation of average stroke volume has been determined during a given time period (often 1 minute), this information can be used in conjunction with knowledge of heart rate across the same time period to determine cardiac output.

Total Peripheral Resistance

Total peripheral resistance of the systemic vasculature is of considerable importance because it is one of the two primary determinants of blood pressure, the other being cardiac output. The simultaneous measurement of blood pressure and cardiac output (CO) makes it possible to derive total peripheral resistance (TPR) from the formula:

$$TPR = MAP/CO$$

Total peripheral resistance is most often reported in units of dyne − sec × cm^{-5}, derived as follows (Sherwood, 1993):

$$TPR(dyne - sec \times cm^{-5}) = [MAP\ (mmHg)/CO\ (lpm)] \times 80$$

Alternatively, it can be presented in units called *peripheral resistance units*.[2] In this case, the computation is:

$$TPR(pru) = MAP(mmHg)/CO\ (lpm)/16.67$$

Defining Reactivity

We shall consider two aspects of the definition of reactivity, namely computational and conceptual.

Computational Definition

In the experimental paradigm employed by much of the research presented in this volume, subjects visit the laboratory and perform one or more standardized tasks. Physiological recording takes place during the task itself and also during another period when the subject is asked simply to relax as much as possible. Investigators subsequently use baseline values and task values, also called *task absolute levels*, of a particular variable to calculate a change score. The most commonly used representation of change is the arithmetic difference between the task level and the baseline value. The resultant value is the *reactivity score*. Thus, for heart rate, for example

Heart rate reactivity = Task heart rate minus Baseline heart rate.

It is true that there are other ways of representing a given change in physiological activity. One of these involves the calculation of percentage change from baseline to task. Hence, a baseline of 70 bpm and a task level of 105 bpm would yield a reactivity score of 35 bpm and a percentage change score of 50%. However, it is also true that much of the

---

[2]For discussion of the units of total peripheral resistance, see Guyton, 1981, p. 212.

research described in this volume employed simple arithmetic differences between task levels and baseline levels to calculate reactivity scores, a strategy endorsed by many authors (e.g., Llabre *et al.*, 1991; Pickering, 1991b).

It should be noted at this point that the seemingly simple job of obtaining an appropriate baseline is more complex than it first appears. Knowing that one is about to engage in a stressful situation can itself influence physiological activity. Heart rates of athletes waiting for competitive track events to start were dramatically elevated above resting levels (McArdle *et al.*, 1967). In addition, heart rates were elevated more immediately prior to a short race (an average of 148 bpm) than prior to a 2-mile event (an average of 108 bpm). The fact that the rapid start of vigorous activity is much more important in a sprint event suggests that the greater heart rate elevations prior to that event were at least partly due to anticipatory psychological arousal (Sherwood & Turner, 1992).

Anticipatorily mediated cardiovascular increases have also been described in the psychophysiological laboratory (see Obrist & Light, 1988; Turner & Carroll, 1985a). While this phenomenon is of interest in itself, since this volume focuses on psychological influences on cardiovascular activity, it can also be problematic in the calculation of change scores. An elevated baseline and a given task level will lessen the computed reactivity score. Because of the possibility that baseline periods held immediately before the stressor may be influenced by anticipation, some investigators have chosen another time to use as a baseline period (either sometime after task completion, or at the same time of day on a separate day). If a pretask baseline period is used, a procedure which is commonly adopted, a period of relaxation of between 15 and 30 minutes has been recommended (see Hastrup, 1986; Schneiderman & McCabe, 1989).

Conceptual Definition

The computational definition given above allows the calculation of reactivity for one variable at a time, and it is obviously very important and necessary. However, in some ways, the computational definition can be better regarded as defining a *response*, rather than defining reactivity. In the larger sense of the word "reactivity," there is much more to the concept than this simple calculation of a difference score (i.e., a response) for any one variable. Sherwood recently provided a more rigorous definition (Sherwood & Turner, 1992, p. 3):

> Cardiovascular reactivity is a psychophysiological construct referring to the magnitude, patterns, and/or mechanisms of cardiovascular responses associated with exposure to psychological stress. It is a term that is used to refer to the propensity for an individual to exhibit an alteration in cardiovascular activity during exposure to some external, predominantly psychological stimulus, which may, or may not, elicit an active behavioral response.

This definition highlights two important points. First, while very informative studies examining only one cardiovascular parameter can certainly be conducted, current interest often focuses on the *pattern* of concurrent alteration seen in several variables. Second, the word "propensity" indicates that what we are ultimately looking for here is a *consistent tendency* of an individual to show large (or small) responses to given, relevant stimuli, which may indicate a greater (or lesser) risk for cardiovascular disease. Encapsulated within these two points are the major foci of this volume, which addresses the hypothesized trilateral stress-reactivity-disease connection.

Hemodynamic Patterning

As just noted, response patterns are now attracting a lot of experimental attention. Of particular interest is *hemodynamic patterning*. Cardiac output and total peripheral resistance of the systemic vasculature, as noted earlier, are the underlying hemodynamic determinants of blood pressure. Because blood pressure (BP) is the figurative and mathematical product of these two variables (i.e., BP = CO × TPR), an increase in blood pressure can be the result of a change in cardiac output, a change in total peripheral resistance, or a change in both. It should be noted here that a large increase in one of these variables can still lead to an overall increase in blood pressure even if the other variable shows a decrease. Consider the following equation:

$$4 \times 3 = 12$$

If we *increase* the 4 to 10, and *decrease* the 3 to 2, the equation now reads:

$$10 \times 2 = 20$$

The product of these variables has increased considerably, from 12 to 20, even though one of the variables actually decreased.

It is also of considerable interest to note that in the above example the same degree of change (i.e., an increase of 8, from 12 to 20) can be achieved in various ways by different combinations of changes in the two variables. Moving back from this mathematical example to real blood pressure issues, the fascinating opportunity afforded by the measurement of the underlying hemodynamic determinants is the ascertainment of whether a given blood pressure change is primarily a function of a change in cardiac output or a change in total peripheral resistance. This determination is of great interest in terms of differing stressors, and also in terms of both individual subjects and groups of subjects. We shall consider these in turn.

A Classification System for Stressors

One way of classifying different stressors is to look at the hemo- dynamic response patterns that they evoke in subjects. Early studies employing impedance cardiography in reactivity paradigms in this manner revealed that different stressors affect the cardiac and vascular deter- minants of blood pressure in different ways (Lovallo *et al.*, 1985, 1986a, b).

Table 3.1 presents mean data collected from 36 subjects during a reaction time task and a cold pressor task (see Turner *et al.*, 1991). Presented are mean baseline data, mean task levels, and mean reactivity scores. It can be seen from the figures in Table 3.1 that the equation "reactivity = task level minus baseline" can be used for group mean levels as well as for an individual subject's data. Using mean baseline and mean task levels in this fashion to obtain mean reactivity scores is

Table 3.1. Mean Absolute Values and Reactivity Scores for SBP, DBP, CO, and TPR (n = 36) for Reaction Time and Cold Pressor[a]

	SBP (mmHg)	DBP (mmHg)	CO (l/m)	TPR (dyne − sec × cm^{-5})
Absolute values				
Baseline	124	81	4.55	1830
Reaction time	142	87	6.25	1582
Cold pressor	144	95	4.63	2216
Reactivity scores				
Reaction time	18	6	1.70	−248
Cold pressor	20	14	0.08	386

Adapted from J.R. Turner, A. Sherwood, & K.C. Light, 1991.
[a]SBP = Systolic blood pressure; DBP = Diastolic blood pressure; CO = Cardiac output; TPR = Total peripheral resistance.

mathematically equivalent to calculating reactivity scores separately for each individual in the group and then taking the mean of the individual reactivity scores.

Both tasks elicited blood pressure increases, and the systolic increases were particularly similar. However, in the case of the reaction time task, blood pressure increases were mediated by a large increase in cardiac output (total peripheral resistance falling), whereas blood pressure increases during the cold pressor were mediated primarily by an increase in total peripheral resistance (coupled with a very slight increase in cardiac output). These two tasks thus display very different hemodynamic patterning. The reaction time task might therefore be regarded as a "cardiac" task, whereas the cold pressor might be regarded as a "vascular" task.

This task-classification system, therefore, is one which groups tasks according to which hemodynamic determinant is primarily responsible for the blood pressure responses that the task elicits. Another way of expressing this is by considering the mechanisms leading to the differing hemodynamic patterns in question. Thus, the relative contribution of alpha-adrenergic and beta-adrenergic mechanisms of cardiovascular stress responses has itself become a widely used classification system for identifying and describing types of stressors (Sherwood & Turner, 1992). The reaction time task is a good example of a beta-adrenergic task, since it elicits blood pressure increases largely mediated by increased cardiac output. On the other hand, the cold pressor task is a good example of an alpha-adrenergic task, since it elicits blood pressure increases primarily via its vasoconstrictive effects, which are mediated by alpha-adrenergic receptor stimulation.

This system of task classification circumvents the classification problems of the physical/psychological and active/passive systems discussed earlier. Placing a task into one of the categories in this hemodynamic patterning system can be done more objectively. If the physiological responses to a given task are monitored for a large group of subjects, it will become apparent which hemodynamic pattern that task typically elicits.

Individual Differences in Hemodynamic Patterning

The penultimate word in the previous section—i.e., "typically"—is important. It hints at one of the key foci of interest in this volume. A given task (or situation) does not *always* elicit the same response from *all* individuals. That is, there are *individual differences* in response patterns during stress. Instead of this being a nuisance, in that everyone does not react in the same manner, it is actually an extremely important occurrence from the researcher's point of view.

Imagine a scenario where, during a stressor, two individuals show similarly sizable increases in blood pressure. Until recently, these two individuals would, quite logically, have been considered to have reacted in the same manner. However, it is possible that the first person's blood pressure alterations were mediated primarily by an increase in cardiac output, whereas the second person's blood pressure responses were mediated primarily by an increase in total peripheral resistance. In fact, this scenario is more than possible; it can be seen in real data.

Figure 3.1 shows data from two subjects in an experiment by Dr. Andrew Sherwood and colleagues at the University of North Carolina at Chapel Hill. The two subjects, A and B, were among a group of subjects who completed a mental arithmetic task. Their blood pressure responses were very similar. However, examination of the underlying hemodynamic determinants of these blood pressure responses indicated that for Subject A, cardiac output increased significantly, whereas peripheral resistance actually decreased slightly; in contrast, Subject B showed an increase in vascular resistance coupled with minimal alteration in cardiac output.

One feature of the phenomenon of individual differences in cardiovascular reactivity is that it allows individual subjects within a group to be placed in reactor subgroups. For example, the half (or the third, or quarter, perhaps) of subjects showing the greatest heart rate reactivity during a stressor might be placed into the High Heart Rate Reactor Group, whereas the commensurate number of individuals showing the least reactivity would be placed into the Low Heart Rate Reactor Group. This creation of reactor groups can be done on the basis of responses of any one variable. However, in a more sophisticated and informative manner, consideration of the hemodynamic patterning shown by individual subjects allows subgroups to be formed on this basis. Thus, two reactor subgroups that might be formed are Vascular Reactors and Cardiac Reactors. These consist of individual subjects who primarily mediate their blood pressure responses during stress by vascular (total peripheral resistance) and cardiac (cardiac output) routes, respectively. Individual differences in cardiovascular reactivity (both magnitude of response and underlying hemodynamic patterning) will be considered in detail in Chapter 5.

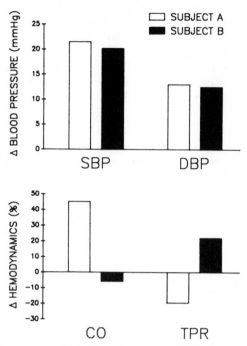

Figure 3.1. Systolic pressure (SBP), diastolic pressure (DBP), cardiac output (CO), and vascular resistance (TPR) responses to a mental arithmetic task in two individuals displaying contrasting hemodynamic mechanisms underlying similar blood pressure responses. Reprinted with permission from Sherwood & Turner, 1992. New York: © Plenum Press.

Group Differences in Hemodynamic Patterning

In the previous section we saw how a collection of individuals can be placed into different groups according to their individual reactivity. This is one strategy commonly employed in reactivity research. A second strategy is to start with two (or more) groups of subjects formed according to another criterion (for example, male and female gender groups), and then to examine the reactivity typically displayed by members of these groups. Examination of adult gender groups, for example generally shows that men show greater overall systolic blood pressure responses than do women (see Chapter 8, which focuses on group differences in reactivity). Another example of this strategy concerns the comparison of physiological responses shown by African

Americans and Caucasian Americans. This example is particularly pertinent in this discussion of hemodynamic patterning, since these groups differ in this regard. Relative to Caucasian Americans, African Americans tend to mediate their blood pressure responses to psycho-physiological stressors more via the vascular route than via the cardiac route (see Anderson *et al.*, 1992; also see Chapter 8 of this text).

Before leaving this section on group differences in hemodynamic patterning, it should be emphasized that individual variations will exist within these (or any other such) groups. For example, there will be individual women who show blood pressure responses greater than those shown by many men, and there will be Caucasian Americans who mediate their blood pressure responses via the vascular route.

Summary

Stress causes a spectacular pattern of cardiovascular-hormonal change called the *fight-or-flight response*. Stress can be modeled in the laboratory using psychological stressors, which engage and stimulate subjects. Examples of such stressors are reaction time tasks, mental arithmetic, and video games.

Reactivity refers to the magnitude, patterns, and/or mechanisms of cardiovascular responses associated with exposure to psychological stress. Computationally, it is defined as "task level minus baseline level." The responses of variables such as heart rate, blood pressure, cardiac output, and total peripheral resistance can therefore be considered individually. However, it can be more informative to consider *patterns* of response. Because blood pressure is determined by the hemodynamic variables of cardiac output and total peripheral resistance, the same blood pressure increase can be the result of various combinations of alterations in these underlying hemodynamic variables. The responses typically elicited by a specific task, and the responses typically displayed by an individual or a group of subjects during stress, can be classified using different hemodynamic response pattern categories.

Further Reading

1. Julius S. (1989). Hemodynamic assessment and pharmacologic probes as tools to analyze cardiovascular reactivity. In N. Schneiderman, S.M. Weiss, & P.G. Kaufmann

(Eds.), *Handbook of research methods in cardiovascular behavioral medicine* (pp. 411–416). New York: Plenum.

2. Light, K.C. (1981). Cardiovascular responses to effortful active coping: Implications for the role of stress in hypertension development. *Psychophysiology, 18*, 216–225.

3. Obrist, P.A. (1976). The cardiovascular–behavioral interaction as it appears today. *Psychophysiology, 13*, 95–107.

4. Schneiderman, N., & McCabe, P.M. (1989). Psychophysiological strategies in laboratory research. In N. Schneiderman, S.M. Weiss, & P.G. Kaufmann (Eds.), *Handbook of research methods in cardiovascular behavioral medicine* (pp. 349–364). New York: Plenum.

5. Sherwood, A. (1993). Use of impedance cardiography in cardiovascular reactivity research. In J. Blascovich & E.S. Katkin (Eds.), *Cardiovascular reactivity to psychological stress and disease* (pp. 157–199). Washington, DC: American Psychological Association.

6. Sherwood, A., Allen, M.T., Fahrenberg, J., Kelsey, R.M., Lovallo, W.R., & van Doornen, L.J.P. (1990). Committee report: Methodological guidelines for impedance cardiography. *Psychophysiology, 27*, 1–23.

7. Sherwood, A., & Turner, J.R. (1992). A conceptual and methodological overview of cardiovascular reactivity research. In J.R. Turner, A. Sherwood, & K.C. Light (Eds.), *Individual differences in cardiovascular response to stress* (pp. 3–32). New York: Plenum.

8. Steptoe, A. (1980). Blood pressure. In I. Martin & P.H. Venables (Eds.), *Techniques in psychophysiology* (pp. 247–273). Chichester: Wiley.

9. Turner, J.R., Hewitt, J.K., Morgan, R.K., Sims, J., Carroll, D., & Kelly, K.A. (1986). Graded mental arithmetic as an active psychological challenge. *International Journal of Psychophysiology,3*, 307–309.

10. Wilson, M.F., Lovallo, W.R., & Pincomb, G.A. (1989). Noninvasive measurement of cardiac functions. In N. Schneiderman, S.M. Weiss, & P.G. Kaufmann (Eds.), *Handbook of research methods in cardiovascular behavioral medicine* (pp. 23–50). New York: Plenum.

CHAPTER 4

Hypertension: The Disease and the Possible Influence of Stress Responses in Its Development

In this final chapter of the book's first section we shall consider the possible association between heightened cardiovascular reactivity and later cardiovascular disease. This potential association has been a major driving force behind reactivity research in recent years, and a considerable number of publications have addressed this issue in detail. Presented here is a selection of the vast quantity of information relating to the role of stress and reactivity in the development of hypertension.

Hypertension

A precise and universally accepted definition of hypertension is difficult to find. Indeed, Folkow and Neil (1971) noted that "disagreements between authorities have often reached levels which cannot be good for their own blood pressure." Julius (1977b) provided some useful guidelines, considering pressures below 140 mmHg/90 mmHg to be "normotensive" and pressures equal to or above 160 mmHg/100 mmHg to be unambiguously "hypertensive." However, more recently there has been an increasing tendency to describe blood pressures between 150 mmHg/90 mmHg and 160 mmHg/100 mmHg as excessively high (Carroll, 1992).

The term *borderline hypertension* has been used to describe two conditions falling somewhere between normotension and hypertension. The first is one in which the blood pressure is constantly elevated, but not sufficiently to be considered "hypertensive." The second concerns blood pressure that fluctuates between normotensive and hypertensive levels. Hence, borderline hypertension, which Julius (1977a) called the "gray zone" between normotension and hypertension, is characterized by moderate elevation and/or by lability.

Blood pressure does not have to reach a specified level before it becomes of concern; any elevation at all is undesirable. The results of various studies have indicated that as blood pressure increases, so life expectancy decreases (Carroll, 1984). Evidence to this effect came from the Framingham Heart Study, a major prospective cardiovascular study of over 5,000 individuals; Kannel and Sorlie (1975, p. 557) commented that

> Compared to "normotensives," "hypertensive" persons develop a marked excess of the major cardiovascular diseases. In the age group 45–74, they develop at least twice as much occlusive peripheral arterial disease, about three times as much coronary disease, more than four times as much congestive failure and over seven times the incidence of brain infarction as do normotensives.

Evidence like this, combined with the statistic that hypertension affects 60 million people in the United States alone (Kannel & Thom, 1986), makes it very clear that hypertension is a major medical concern.

The Development of Hypertension

Throughout this book, the term *hypertension* is used to refer to the condition whose proper name is *essential hypertension*.[1] Essential hypertension is high blood pressure where there is no detectable medical cause or organ pathology. This is the situation in the vast majority of cases of hypertension, but not in all cases. In a small percentage of cases, factors such as renal conditions cause the high blood pressure. Henceforth, we shall focus on essential hypertension.

---

[1]It was once thought that aging inevitably led to atherosclerosis and that elevation of blood pressure was "essential" in order to perfuse blood adequately through body tissues supplied by narrowed atherosclerotic arteries. Irvine Page, who was "the world's foremost pioneer in hypertension research," was "the first to challenge and debunk" this concept (Manger, 1991, p. 197).

The mechanisms underlying hypertension development are likely to be varied and complex (Guyton, 1977b; Page, 1977). However, while acknowledging that there are many controversies concerning these mechanisms, Folkow (1982) pointed out that nearly all authorities would agree on the importance of cardiac factors. This observation explains why there have been hypotheses put forward suggesting that cardiac, and cardiovascular, reactions to psychological stress may play a role in the development of hypertension, or more precisely in the initiation and early stages of its development. Before introducing two of these theories linking cardiovascular reactivity and hypertension, it is appropriate to consider the usual stages in the development of hypertension.

Before the occurrence of full-blown hypertension, individuals may well display borderline hypertension. Borderline hypertension may represent a transitional phase from a normotensive to a hypertensive state (Lovallo & Wilson, 1992b). Borderline hypertensives are at three to four times the risk of normotensives for developing hypertension (Levy et al., 1945), and over time 20% are likely to progress to fixed hypertension (Julius, 1986).

Frohlich et al. (1970) found that individuals with borderline hypertension demonstrated evidence of a condition called "hyperkinetic circulation." This condition is characterized by increased heart rate and cardiac output. Similarly, Lund-Johansen (1983) showed that young borderline hypertensives had elevated cardiac output. Their vascular resistance was found to be normal. Although it is true that not all borderline hypertensives conform to this pattern (see Julius et al., 1975), borderline hypertensives are frequently characterized as displaying an elevated cardiac output and a normal peripheral resistance.

An important point to note is that this hemodynamic pattern changes with the occurrence of full-blown, or sustained, hypertension. Lund-Johansen (1983) reported that, following a 10-year follow-up period of borderline hypertensives displaying the characteristic pattern of elevated cardiac output and normal peripheral resistance, this hemodynamic pattern was reversed. By then, cardiac output was normal and vascular resistance was elevated (see also Lund-Johansen, 1967, 1977). Lund-Johansen's data, therefore, offer evidence that early hypertension can develop over time into a state more typical of sustained hypertension—that is, a state of elevated blood pressure caused by elevated peripheral resistance.

Links between Reactivity and Hypertension

It is important to make clear at the outset that no definitive evidence links high cardiovascular reactivity with hypertension. However, it should also be stated that several lines of evidence, when considered together, suggest inferentially that associations may exist between reactivity and hypertension, and which therefore encourage continued research.

Theories of Hypertension Development

Autoregulation Theory

Both Guyton and colleagues and Obrist and colleagues have expounded the theory that excessive cardiac output may lead to, or be an initiating influence in, the development of hypertension (e.g., Coleman et al., 1971; Guyton et al., 1970; Obrist, 1981; Obrist et al., 1983). Certain psychological stressors can lead to large increases in cardiac output (see Chapters 5 and 6). These increases occur in conjunction with very little additional metabolic demand. This situation is quite different from the increases in cardiac activity that accompany physical exercise. In that case, increases in heart rate and cardiac output occur precisely because of the considerably elevated metabolic demand.

The occurrence of metabolically exaggerated cardiac output increases during psychological stress leads to overperfusion of body tissues, particularly skeletal muscle tissues, with oxygenated blood. Although body tissues do not like having too little oxygen for concurrent demands, they also do not like having too much. In response to the excessive supply of oxygen caused by the increased flow of blood, autoregulatory changes occur that counteract the condition of overperfusion. Arterioles begin to constrict, raising arterial resistance. This increased resistance means that cardiac output is reduced and returns virtually to normal. However, the elevated blood pressure that was initially the result of increased cardiac output persists, except that it is now maintained by an increase in resistance. In this manner, a temporary overshoot in cardiac output can lead to quite a protracted elevation in blood pressure (Obrist, 1976).

Two studies of relevance here are those reported by Forsyth (1971) and by Carroll et al. (1990). Both document changing hemodynamic patterns underlying sustained blood pressure elevations, with evidence being provided from nonhuman and human subjects, respectively. Forsyth (1971) exposed monkeys to 72 hours of continuous work on a shock-avoidance schedule. Mean arterial blood pressure during the baseline period was 102 mmHg. Measurements were taken again after 20 minutes, 4 hours, 24 hours, and 72 hours. The mean values on these occasions were 128 mmHg, 123 mmHg, 125 mmHg, and 123 mmHg, respectively. Sustained significant elevations in blood pressure were thus observed. Mean cardiac output and total peripheral resistance measurements were also made at each of the above time points. Cardiac output was considerably above baseline at the 20-minute mark, but it then fell sequentially across the other time points, returning to just below baseline by 72 hours. Total peripheral resistance, however, showed the opposite pattern of change. It initially fell below baseline, and then rose sequentially to be considerably above baseline by 72 hours. The sustained blood pressure increases were thus initially supported by an increase in cardiac output, but later they were due to an increase in total peripheral resistance.

Carroll *et al.* (1990) presented similar evidence using human subjects, although on this occasion the time frame was much shorter. Subjects in this study completed a 16-minute mental arithmetic task. Again, evidence of a shifting hemodynamic pattern was seen. Blood pressure elevations were initially supported by cardiac output increases, and later supported by total peripheral resistance increases. The authors interpreted these observations as possibly reflecting the physiological effects of autoregulation (Carroll *et al.*, 1990).

Although it may not be the primary stimulus for an increase in blood pressure, increased resistance can maintain elevated blood pressure once it has occurred. If an individual responds to psychological stress with large cardiac increases, and if such stress occurs repeatedly, such an individual may demonstrate sustained blood pressure elevations that lead, over time, to the resetting of blood pressure at a higher level. This resetting of pressure is associated with secondary changes, such as the resetting of arterial baroreceptors.

Carotid baroreceptors are stretch receptors that are sensitive to arterial pressure, and they are located in the carotid sinus in the neck. They are part of a feedback loop called the *carotid sinus reflex*. Baroreceptors want to ensure an even supply of oxygen (and hence blood) to the brain. Both short-term and long-term activity of baroreceptors are important. In the short-term, when they detect a change in blood pressure (a change in pressure on the walls of the carotid sinus), they influence cardiac activity in such a way as to restore pressure to its usual level. For example, immediately upon standing, there is a drop in blood pressure. This is detected by the baroreceptors, and a message is sent to the "cardiac acceleration center" in the medulla (Andreassi, 1989). Increased heart rate then helps to raise blood pressure back to the desired level. On the other hand, and of more relevance for present concerns, when baroreceptors detect an increase in pressure, one way to get pressure back down to the desired level is to decrease cardiac activity. With regard to long-term changes, over time the baroreceptors can become reset, so that the pressure they work to maintain is a higher level of pressure than it was initially. (See Chapleau *et al.*, 1989, and Krieger, 1989, for further discussions of baroreceptor function.)

Structural Adaptation

As blood pressure increases toward hypertensive levels, both the heart and the blood vessels change because of the elevated pressure (Folkow, 1990). Both the blood vessels and the heart, particularly the left ventricle, display hypertrophy. Folkow (1990; see also Folkow, 1982) has described this process of structural adaptation in detail, and the reader is directed to his work and also to the biobehavioral model of hypertension development presented by Lovallo and Wilson (1992a).

Certain individuals may be genetically predisposed to show structural adaptation early in their lives. The technique of echocardiography can be used to measure the dimensions of the heart noninvasively. Schieken *et al.* (1981) have shown that 12-year-olds with high blood pressure display increased left-ventricular mass (hypertrophy). The structural adaptations in the heart and blood vessels, which have often been thought of as the *result* of hypertension, may actually be involved in the development of the disease (see Lovallo & Wilson, 1992a).

One of the consequences of these adaptations is that a given amount of autonomic nervous stimulation will give rise to greater cardiovascular reactions. This is what Folkow refers to as *structural hyperresponsivity*. Greater responsivity causes higher blood pressures during stress. These higher pressures then lead to further structural adaptation, and a positive feedback loop is created in which structural adaptations lead to higher pressures, which in turn initiate further structural modification (Lovallo & Wilson, 1992a). This process leads to a state of sustained hypertension.

We noted above that certain individuals may be genetically predisposed to structural adaptation. Normotensive adolescents who have either one or two hypertensive parents have been shown to have significant cardiac hypertrophy in comparison to normotensive adolescents with normotensive parents (Alli *et al.*, 1990). Family history of hypertension is a topic that has received a lot of attention in this research area (see next section), and the offspring of hypertensives have been shown to carry a substantially greater risk for hypertension development than do the offspring of normotensives. Interestingly, these offspring of hypertensives display structural adaptation relatively early in their lives.

Study of High-Risk Groups

Both of the theories discussed above, which hypothesize links between reactivity and hypertension development, lead to the observation that *if* high reactivity plays a role, it is likely to exert its influence in the early stages of the disease's development. Later on in the progression of the disease, other alterations in the cardiovascular system will have occurred, and these will make it much harder to examine the potential role of reactivity caused by autonomic nervous system responses to psychological stress. Accordingly, we need to study hypertension at its inception, before the development of impairments to the system (Julius & Esler, 1975). A good strategy, therefore, is to study individuals at high risk of becoming hypertensive, but prior to the development of significant structural modification. Two groups of individuals who are particularly informative in this context are borderline hypertensives and individuals with a parental history of hypertension.

Borderline Hypertensives

As already noted, borderline hypertensives are at three to four times the risk of developing sustained hypertension, as compared with normotensives (Levy *et al.*, 1945). Two points concerning this group are in order. First, certain psychological stressors cause, in some highly reactive individuals, a hemodynamic pattern that is very similar to that seen in borderline hypertensives at rest. Because borderline hypertensives are at enhanced risk for hypertension, a legitimate inferential argument suggests that these reactive individuals may also be at risk.

Second, a number of studies have shown that borderline hypertensives display larger cardiovascular reactivity than do normotensives during mental stress tests (e.g., Drummond, 1983; Nestel, 1969; Steptoe *et al.*, 1984). For example, Steptoe and colleagues found that subjects who showed transiently high blood pressures at screening displayed significantly higher heart rate reactions during a video game than did normotensive control subjects. The authors interpreted their results as suggesting that exaggerated cardiac responsiveness may be a characteristic of the prehypertensive profile.

A recent review (Fredrikson & Matthews, 1990) addressed in considerable detail the association between cardiovascular responses to behavioral stress and hypertension. The researchers employed meta-analysis (a statistical procedure that enables the results from disparate studies to be combined) to investigate the blood pressure and heart rate responses to behavioral stress of three groups and their controls: essential hypertensives, borderline hypertensives, and offspring of hypertensives. Relative to normotensive control subjects, the borderline hypertensives showed moderately large and more reliable blood pressure and heart rate responses. Interestingly, this was predominantly the case during stressors "requiring an active behavioral response" (Fredrikson & Matthews, 1990).

This finding was in contrast to that for essential hypertensives. Relative to normotensives, the essential hypertensives also displayed large blood pressure responses, but their responses were more consistently different during "passive stressors, which do not require a behavioral response, than during active stressors" (Fredrikson & Matthews, 1990). Thus, while tasks such as the cold pressor elicit larger responses from essential hypertensives than from controls, differentiation between borderline hypertensives and controls requires the use of stressors containing an active psychological element.

Finally, recent studies that have addressed the hemodynamic determinants of the blood pressure responses shown by borderline hypertensives are relevant. Carroll, Harris, and Cross (1991) assessed hemodynamic adjustments during mental arithmetic in both normotensives and subjects with mildly elevated blood pressure. The groups did not differ reliably in total peripheral resistance, leading the authors to conclude that the relatively high blood pressure of the borderline hypertensive group during the psychological stressor was largely attributable to cardiac output adjustments (Carroll *et al.*, 1991). Sherwood,

Royal, and Light (1993) also found that young male adults with borderline hypertension responded to active coping stressors with greater increases in blood pressure than did normotensive controls. Total peripheral resistance responses were again comparable between the two groups, while the borderline hypertensives showed greater cardiac output increases than did the normotensives. Increased cardiac output, therefore, produced the higher blood pressure responses in the borderline hypertensives (Sherwood *et al.*, 1993). These observations are particularly interesting in light of our earlier discussion of autoregulation as a possible mechanism in hypertension development.

Offspring of Hypertensives

Compared with individuals who have normotensive parents, persons who have hypertensive parents have twice the risk of developing hypertension (Hunt *et al.*, 1986; Stamler *et al.*, 1971). There has been considerable investigation of the relative reactivity shown by persons with a positive parental history of hypertension and those with a negative parental history of the disease. This evidence is discussed in detail in Chapter 7, which focuses on genetic and environmental determinants of individual differences in reactivity. For now, we can simply note that considerable evidence shows that the offspring of hypertensives display greater reactivity than do the offspring of normotensives (although it should be noted that such evidence comes predominantly from studies employing Caucasian subjects; see Anderson *et al.*, 1992). As was noted in the previous section, Fredrikson & Matthews (1990) also examined in their review the responses of offspring of hypertensives. They concluded that members of this risk group show elevated systolic blood pressure and heart rate responses to both active and passive stressors, and elevated diastolic blood pressure responses to active stressors. Once again, it appears that active psychological stressors are necessary to reveal the full extent of differences in the cardiovascular responses of normotensives and members of risk groups.

Implications of Evidence from High-Risk Groups

The evidence just reviewed suggests a possible association between reactivity and hypertension, and it strongly encourages continued investigation into the nature of this association. However, it must be made clear that evidence of an association is not sufficient to show that reactivity plays a *causal role* in hypertension development. It may simply be that those who eventually develop hypertension also display heightened reactivity during earlier years. In this case, rather than reactivity being a mechanism in the development of hypertension, it may serve as a marker; that is, it might help in identifying those who go on to develop hypertension even though it is in no way responsible for the development of the disease. Far from being uninteresting and unimportant, the identification of reactivity as a marker, even if it is not a mechanism, would itself be very useful when trying to predict the development of later hypertension (a topic discussed in Chapter 10).

These two models of the association between heightened cardiovascular reactivity and essential hypertension have been referred to as the "mechanism" and "marker" models (e.g., Alpert & Wilson, 1992), and also as the "direct cause" and "risk marker" models (Manuck *et al.*, 1990). Manuck *et al.* (1990) also presented two other possible models, called the "diathesis-stress" model and the "effect modification" model. The diathesis-stress model examines the interaction between vulnerabilities (biological predispositions to react in a given, potentially deleterious, manner) of the individual and the demands of the social environment in which that individual functions. A person who is highly disposed to show heightened reactivity during stressful situations will only do so if such situations are actually encountered.

The effect modification model examines how variables "may often exert a synergistic influence on disease," such that "the relative influence of one risk factor varies in a non-additive fashion with the presence or absence of a second risk variable" (Manuck *et al.*, 1990, p. 27). For further details about these models, the reader is strongly encouraged to read Manuck and colleagues' (1990) account of them, and their respective support, limitations, and implications.

Although these models differ in various ways from each other, they share a common element. All of them examine ways in which individual differences in cardiovascular response to stress might be related to hypertension. Therefore, the next step in our examination of cardiovascular reactivity and stress is to investigate the phenomenon of individual differences in reactivity. Accordingly, it is to a detailed examination of these individual differences that we shall now turn.

Summary

Hypertension is a prevalent disease. In most cases it occurs with no detectable medical or organic cause. Hypothesized links between reactivity and hypertension have been suggested, and theories such as autoregulation theory and structural adaptation have been put forward. Reactivity may play a role in the development of hypertension, or it may occur in those who eventually develop the disease while playing no role in its development. In the latter case, reactivity would be a marker (as opposed to a mechanism in the former case) for disease development. Confirmation of reactivity as either a mechanism or a marker would be very important in predicting later disease.

Further Reading

1. Folkow, B. (1990). "Structural factor" in primary and secondary hypertension. *Hypertension, 16*, 89–101.
2. Folkow, B., & Neil, E. (1971). *Circulation*. New York: Oxford University Press.
3. Fredrikson, M., & Matthews, K.A. (1990). Cardiovascular responses to behavioral stress and hypertension: A meta-analytic review. *Annals of Behavioral Medicine, 12*, 30–39.
4. Genest, J., Koiw, E., & Kuchel, O. (1977). *Hypertension: Pathophysiology and treatment*. New York: McGraw-Hill.
5. Kannel, W.B., & Sorlie, P. (1975). Hypertension in Framingham. In O. Paul (Ed.), *Epidemiology and control of hypertension* (pp. 553–592). New York: Intercontinental Medical Book Corporation.
6. Lovallo, W.R., & Wilson, M.F. (1992). A biobehavioral model of hypertension development. In J.R. Turner, A. Sherwood, & K.C. Light (Eds.), *Individual differences in cardiovascular response to stress* (pp. 265–280). New York: Plenum.
7. Manuck, S.B., Kasprowicz, A.L., & Muldoon, M.F. (1990). Behaviorally-evoked cardiovascular reactivity and hypertension: Conceptual issues and potential associations. *Annals of Behavioral Medicine, 12*, 17–29.
8. Matthews, K.A., Weiss, S.M., Detre, T., Dembroski, T.M., Falkner, B., Manuck, S.B., & Williams, R.B., Jr. (1986). *Handbook of stress, reactivity, and cardiovascular disease*. New York: Wiley.
9. Obrist, P.A. (1985). Beta-adrenergic hyperresponsivity to behavioral challenges: A possible hypertensive risk factor. In J.F. Orlebeke, G. Mulder, & L.J.P. van Doornen (Eds.), *Psychophysiology of cardiovascular control: Methods, models, and data* (pp. 667–682). New York: Plenum.
10. Steptoe, A. (1981). *Psychological factors in cardiovascular disorders*. London: Academic Press.

PART II

Laboratory Investigation of
Cardiovascular Reactivity

Chapter 5

Individual Differences in Cardiovascular Reactivity

The physiological reactions elicited by psychological stress vary in their magnitude and, indeed, patterning, for two main reasons: One is the precise nature of the challenge (the "situational factor") and the other is the nature of the person's biological program (the "individual factor"). While any given response in an individual subject is a function of *both* factors, this chapter will focus on the *individual factor*.

What does this individual factor mean? It says that if we expose a group of subjects to exactly the same situation, there will be a range in the amount of psychophysiological reactivity elicited among members of that group. In other words, there will be individual differences in response. To attribute these differences entirely to the individuals and not the situation, we need to keep the situation completely constant. This is a main goal of experimental laboratory work in any area of psychology or other behavioral science. It is probably fair to say that we can never manage this perfectly, but we must attempt to do so very determinedly. Hence, the physical conditions of the experimental chamber (level of illumination, temperature, humidity, sound attenuation), the experimental task, and the experimental protocol and behavior of all experimenters should be as identical as possible from test session to test session. Only when this is achieved can we reasonably attribute differences in subjects' responses to the Individual Factor.

One practical strategy that can be employed when attempting to ascribe individual differences in reactivity to this individual, or biological, factor is to assess subjects' ratings of a given task. This can be done by asking them, at the end of the task, to place a mark somewhere on a visual-analog scale to indicate how mentally engaged they felt by the task. It is almost certain that there will be some differences between subjects in this regard. However, the important issue here is to examine the relationship between these differences and differences in reactivity. Correlational analysis can be employed here. If there is found to be no significant relationship between subjects' degree of mental engagement by the task and their reactivity scores, individual differences in reactivity cannot be ascribed to differing perceptions of the task. It can, however, be ascribed to differences in the biological factor.

Carroll's group performed such analyses in many studies and found no evidence for a relationship between degree of mental engagement and reactivity (e.g., Turner & Carroll, 1985a). Individual differences in reactivity, therefore, were not simply a function of how engaged subjects were by the task.

The possible influence of task performance on reactivity was similarly investigated. Turner and Carroll (1985a) examined the relationship between reactivity and performance on both video game and mental arithmetic tasks. Both tasks were well suited to objective assessments of performance. For the mental arithmetic task, the number of errors made was used. For the video game, three indices of performance were used: (1) the first points score obtained, (2) the best score obtained, and (3) improvement (the difference between the two former indices). None of the correlation coefficients calculated between performance and reactivity even came close to being statistically significant, revealing that reactivity was not merely a function of the individual's task performance.

These investigations are crucial prerequisites in examining the influence of a biological factor. This evidence suggests that the biological factor does indeed play a role in determining reactivity. Reactivity scores are independent of reported degree of involvement in a task, and of task performance. The degree of reactivity shown by an individual, therefore, appears to be an independent measure of biological propensity to react in a given manner.

Let us now examine some real data to obtain a sense of the range of individual differences seen in cardiovascular responses to psychological stress. Table 5.1 presents heart rate and blood pressure data collected by Sherwood *et al*. (1992a). These examples bear witness to the considerable range of individual differences seen in reactivity to tasks employed

Table 5.1. Mean, Minimum, and Maximum Systolic Blood Pressure (SBP), Diastolic Blood Pressure (DBP), and Heart Rate (HR) Responses to a Series of Laboratory Stressors in 20 Healthy Young Male Adults

Task	Mean	Minimum	Maximum
Mental arithmetic			
SBP (mmHg)	20	5	42
DBP (mmHg)	8	−1	28
HR (bpm)	22	5	47
Reaction time			
SBP (mmHg)	20	−1	41
DBP (mmHg)	3	−9	12
HR (bpm)	19	0	48
Speech stressor			
SBP (mmHg)	32	10	60
DBP (mmHg)	21	6	35
HR (bpm)	25	6	44
Mirror trace			
SBP (mmHg)	11	−5	31
DBP (mmHg)	8	−9	33
HR (bpm)	5	−9	18
Forehead cold pressor			
SBP (mmHg)	20	5	34
DBP (mmHg)	20	8	47
HR (bpm)	−2	−15	16

Reprinted, with permission, from Sherwood & Turner, 1992. New York: ©Plenum Press.

in behavioral medicine paradigms. Presentation of mean values alone conceals this enormous individual variation.

A very important point to make here is that, for present purposes, the individual differences seen are of *much* greater interest than the mean values. Of course, means are informative, but in this context the individual differences are much more so. To illustrate this point, consider the hypothetical data presented in Table 5.2, showing heart rate reactivity scores to two different tasks. Task A elicited a mean increase of 40 bpm, while task B only elicited a mean reactivity score of 20 bpm. It is tempting to think of task A as being "twice as good" since it led to twice as much total reactivity. However, from our point of view, task B is much more informative since the *range of responses* is much greater. For

Table 5.2. Hypothetical Heart Rate
Reactivity Scores during Two Tasks

Task A	Task B
38	20
37	5
39	2
42	10
40	35
43	30
41	16
40	24
44	38
36	20
Mean: 40	Mean: 20

Note: Ten subjects did each task.

task A, this range was only 8 bpm (from 36 bpm to 44 bpm); for task B, the range was 36 bpm.

Often, researchers will split up a group of subjects into High Reactors and Low Reactors, based upon their reactivity scores to a certain task. One way to do this is to use a median split (i.e., simply dividing subjects into two groups by putting the half showing the highest scores into the high reactor group, and the half showing the lowest scores into the low reactor group). Another strategy is to select the top quarter or third, for example, to be the high reactors, and the equivalent number of the lowest individuals to be the low reactor group. In this light, consider the subjects who completed task A. All of these individuals showed very similar responses, all fairly close to the mean reactivity score of 40 bpm. Therefore, if we were to create high and low reactor groups, the difference between these groups would not be very great. However, now consider the subjects who completed task B. The range of individual differences is much greater, and it would be possible to create high and low reactor groups that really did look different from each other.

To emphasize this point, imagine that both tasks A and B were actually completed by the *same* 10 individuals. Using task A would not really allow us to differentiate very well between reactive and nonreactive individuals, whereas using task B would be extremely useful. The next question here is, why do we want to be able to distinguish between high and low reactors? Or, in other words, why do we want to be able to categorize an individual as a high or a low reactor? This simple question and its answer are central to research in this area of cardiovascular behavioral medicine. The answer lies in our investigation of the possible relationship between reactivity and the development of hypertension.

As we saw in the previous chapter, it has been hypothesized that high reactivity may play a causal role in the development of hypertension (e.g., Obrist, 1981). It has also been hypothesized that, even if not causally related, the occurrence of high reactivity in young adulthood may provide a useful marker for the later development of hypertension (e.g., see Manuck et al., 1990). In either case, identification of high reactors is potentially useful in identifying individuals at risk for later hypertension.

Not everyone develops hypertension, so for reactivity to be of any use in prediction there must be individuals who show low reactivity and those who show high reactivity; that is, there must be individual variation. In this context, our tasks should be considered successful if they elicit such individual differences, even if they produce relatively small mean changes. If a task is too easy, it will fail to engage people, and the potential high reactors will be indistinguishable from the low reactors since everyone will show very small changes. Conversely, if a situation is so arousing that every subject shows marked cardiac response, the same identification problem would arise. We must remain aware, therefore, that tasks are simply a means to an end and that our focus must not fixate on specific situations or stressors per se, but on their ability to provide useful information.

When considering current hypotheses linking cardiovascular reactivity to aspects of cardiovascular disease, three attributes of individual differences in reactivity have particular significance (Manuck et al., 1989). These are (1) the temporal stability of individual differences in responses; (2) the reproducibility of these differences in different situations, or during different tasks; and (3) the generalizability of individual differences in responses obtained in the psychophysiological laboratory to measurements made in natural settings in the real world.

Measures of temporal stability assess the degree to which the individual differences seen within a group of subjects on one occasion of testing are similar to those displayed by the same individuals some time later. These measures have most frequently been reported as simple correlation coefficients, depicting the degree of correspondence of reactivity assessed at an initial test session with that at a subsequent test session (Sherwood & Turner, 1992).

Intertask consistency describes consistency of response between different stressors typically encountered in a single experimental session; psychophysiological experiments are increasingly employing several stressors, a strategy strongly endorsed by several prominent authors (e.g., Manuck *et al.*, 1990; Pickering & Gerin, 1990).

Laboratory–real-world generalization, or laboratory-field generalization, concerns the relationship between laboratory stress responses and responses to real-world situations encountered during daily life; it examines the degree to which individual differences in laboratory responses are associated with individual differences in responses during naturalistic stressors. Intertask consistency and laboratory-field generalization can be regarded, both conceptually and descriptively, as two aspects of Situational Stability (Sherwood & Turner, 1992), and as is the case for temporal stability, both are often assessed via simple correlational analyses.

The relevance of these three attributes of individual differences in cardiovascular reactivity to disease states becomes evident from the assertion that the pathogenic influence of large stress-induced responses depends in part on those responses showing reproducibility across time and across different behavioral challenges (Matthews *et al.*, 1987). If excessive cardiovascular adjustments are to be implicated in the etiology of cardiovascular pathology, it is reasonable to argue that a given individual should react in the same way to the same stressor met at different times, and should react similarly to various different stressors. These "different stressors" may be two or more laboratory stressors, or laboratory stressors and real-life stressors. We shall consider temporal stability and intertask consistency in some detail in this chapter. Laboratory-field generalization will be discussed in Chapter 9.

Temporal Stability

Heart Rate and Blood Pressure

Carroll, Turner, and colleagues examined the temporal stability of heart rate reactivity to a video game in several studies, two of which were reported by Carroll *et al.* (1984). In the first of these, 42 subjects completed the video game task on two occasions, exactly one week apart. Each subject completed the tasks at the same time of day on each occasion (to control for any possible influence of circadian rhythm). Heart rate reactivity scores for the two occasions were highly correlated: $r(40) = 0.80$; $p < .01$.

In the second study, 3 extreme high and 3 extreme low reactors were selected from a pool of 23 subjects on the basis of their heart rate reactions during an initial test session. The average reactivity score for the 3 high reactors was $+29.9$ bpm; for the 3 low reactors the mean was -2.0 bpm.[1] These 6 subjects then returned to the laboratory approximately 2 weeks after their initial visits and completed four more testing sessions. These additional sessions took place on consecutive days and, for each subject, were scheduled at the same time of day. Figure 5.1 depicts the mean reactivity scores for each group for both the original session and the four subsequent sessions. All five mean values for the low reactor group are essentially zero; members of this group consistently showed minimal cardiovascular response. In striking contrast, the cardiac impact of the video game on members of the high reactor group was very considerable; the five mean reactivity values were all above 20 bpm. High and low reactivity remained stable features of the respective criterion groups during each occasion of measurement.

These examples have involved only heart rate; what do the data for blood pressure look like? Manuck and Schaefer (1978) tested 42 subjects twice, again a week apart, using a concept formation task. For systolic blood pressure, the correlation coefficient was 0.68, and for diastolic it was 0.46. Manuck and Garland (1980) retested 19 of the original 42 subjects just over a year later. They compared the new reactivity scores

---

[1]It should be noted here that it is mathematically possible to obtain a negative reactivity score. Because reactivity scores are calculated as task level minus baseline level, a negative reactivity score will result if the task level is less than the baseline level. While this certainly does occur in real data every now and then, the occurrence of negative reactivity scores in the type of psychological tasks discussed in this volume is relatively rare for heart rate and blood pressure. And, when they do occur, they are very small in magnitude. Conceptually, these isolated cases can be thought of as indicating no reactivity (i.e., a reactivity score of zero). It should be emphasized, however, that the same is not true for other cardiovascular parameters. Decreases (that is, negative reactivity scores) are of particular interest in some cases. For example, a *decrease* in interbeat interval when a particular stressor is imposed (which is analogous to an increase in heart rate) can be of interest if that index of cardiac function is being used in a given study.

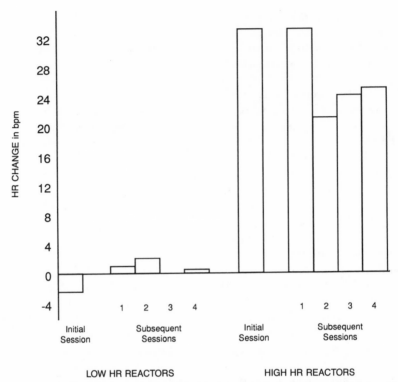

Figure 5.1. Average heart rate (HR) reactivity of high and low reactors. Reprinted, with permission, from Carroll *et al.*, 1984. ©Elsevier Science Publishers B.V. (North-Holland).

with the averages of subjects' reactivity scores from the previous testing and obtained correlation coefficients of 0.63 for systolic blood pressure and 0.24 for diastolic pressure. Manuck and colleagues also measured heart rate on each occasion of testing. The heart rate correlations they obtained were very much in line with those presented earlier; the coefficients were 0.69 for the one-week retest and 0.81 for the one-year retest.

The reliability of systolic blood pressure reactivity across time is relatively impressive in the above studies, but this is not the case for diastolic reactivity. Several authors (e.g., Sherwood & Turner, 1992; Steptoe & Vögele, 1991) have commented on this pattern of findings, which is typical for a large body of literature that now addresses temporal stability. Reasons for the lack of stability for diastolic reactivity may speculatively involve physiological, statistical, and methodological factors. It may be influenced by (1) the dependence upon complex cardiac and vascular interactions determining diastolic pressure responses; (2) the relatively smaller changes in diastolic pressure reported for many behavioral challenges, such that low correlations may be influenced by the relatively restricted ranges of values employed in their calculation; and (3) the comparative difficulty in accurately measuring diastolic pressure compared with heart rate and systolic pressure measurement.

Strikingly similar results to these initial reports have been found by other investigators using a variety of laboratory tasks (e.g., Allen *et al.*, 1987; Lovallo *et al.*, 1986a; Matthews *et al.*, 1987; Van Egeren & Sparrow, 1989). However, agreement has not been unanimous (Arena *et al.*, 1983), and neither has a positive interpretation of the body of literature as a whole. For example, Pickering and Gerin (1990, p. 4) commented that "given the mixed results and the relatively small amount of work done in this area, we conclude that the reliability of cardiovascular reactivity still remains to be demonstrated." These comments, however, followed discussion of only seven studies.

A more recent review examined the data from a much larger group of experiments. Steptoe and Vögele (1991) employed elegant statistical techniques that allow the results from different studies to be combined to produce a representative coefficient, called an *average-weighted correlation coefficient*. Their analysis yielded average-weighted correlation coefficients of 0.62, 0.52, and 0.30 for heart rate reactivity, systolic pressure reactivity, and diastolic reactivity, respectively. These values suggest heart rate and systolic blood pressure reactivity scores display reasonable temporal stability, especially when one considers them in conjunction with evaluations of the temporal stability of baseline values. When baseline values are examined in this manner, temporal stability correlation coefficients seldom exceed 0.75 (Manuck *et al.*, 1989). Therefore, it may be unreasonable to expect reactivity temporal stability coefficients to approach 1.00, since this is not the case for baseline values either. All of these considerations support the view that there is now reasonable evidence of the temporal stability of heart rate and blood pressure responses.

Hemodynamic Variables

Two out of three earlier studies found cardiac output responses to show moderate to good levels of test-retest reliability (McKinney *et al.*,

1985; Myrtek, 1985; cf. Fahrenberg *et al.*, 1985). More recently, following growing interest in the possible pathogenic significance of individual variation in these hemodynamic constituents of cardiovascular reactivity, five studies have evaluated the stability of both cardiac and vascular components of blood pressure responses.

Kasprowicz *et al.* (1990) tested 39 college students on a mental arithmetic and a mirror drawing task; the test-retest interval was 4 weeks. Generally, correlation coefficients showed moderate test-retest reliability for the cardiac and vascular, as well as blood pressure, responses to the tasks. In a further, *post hoc* analysis of their data, Kasprowicz *et al.* (1990) identified well-differentiated subgroups of individuals whose blood pressure responses were primarily due to increased cardiac output and those who showed increased vascular resistance (i.e., cardiac and vascular reactors). Individuals so identified showed impressive temporal stability of the cardiac output and total peripheral resistance adjustments underlying their blood pressure responses.

Sherwood *et al.* (1990c) employed data from a competitive reaction time task to examine the responses of 13 subjects across a 3-month interval. Test-retest correlations were calculated for a number of response measures, including heart rate, systolic and diastolic blood pressure, cardiac output, and total peripheral resistance. The results are presented in Table 5.3. All of the correlations except that for diastolic reactivity attained significance. Moreover, the magnitudes of the cor-

Table 5.3.   Test-Retest Correlation Coefficients
($n = 13$) for Cardiovascular Reactivity
to the Reaction Time Task

Cardiovascular measure	Correlation coefficient
Systolic blood pressure	0.67*
Diastolic blood pressure	0.31
Heart rate	0.91**
Cardiac output	0.81**
Total peripheral resistance	0.70*

*$p < 0.02$.
**$p < 0.001$.
(Adapted from Sherwood, Turner, Light, and Blumenthal, 1990).

relations indicated that the test-retest reliability of cardiac output and total peripheral resistance were at least as good as that evident for blood pressure.

This observation is in line with the conclusion that can be drawn from these and three more recent studies (Kamarck *et al.*, 1992; Llabre *et al.*, 1993; Saab *et al.*, 1992), which is that hemodynamic patterning may be more stable over time than blood pressure reactivity scores themselves (Sherwood & Turner, 1992).

Intertask Consistency

Heart Rate and Blood Pressure

Intertask consistency, as noted earlier, has also typically been investigated using correlation analysis. Such analysis was employed by Manuck and Garland (1980). They found a correlation of 0.86 between heart rate changes during a concept formation task and a serial subtraction mental arithmetic task. For systolic and diastolic blood pressure responses, the correlations were 0.50 and 0.23, respectively. Light (1981) employed two different reaction time tasks (a shock-avoidance version and a direct head-to-head version) and found significant correlations. In a series of experiments conducted by Turner and Carroll (see Turner, 1988, for a review), the intertask consistency of heart rate reactivity during various stressors was explored. The majority of these studies employed a video game task in conjunction with either a mental arithmetic task or a reaction time task. Intertask correlation coefficient magnitude varied in the studies, but a value of 0.4 in one study (Turner *et al.*, 1986a) is not atypical.

Although this coefficient achieved high statistical significance (owing to a large sample size), its magnitude is somewhat less than the heart rate reactivity correlations for test-retest reliability discussed earlier, and also somewhat less than those reported for intertask consistency by Light (1981) and by Manuck and colleagues (Manuck & Garland, 1980; Manuck & Proietti, 1982). An examination of why this might be led Turner (1988) to conclude that the tasks used by Turner and Carroll were more different from each other than those used by Light and by Manuck and colleagues.

This raises an interesting issue. If we are only able to demonstrate intertask consistency when tasks are very similar to each other, evidence of the true existence of such consistency is weakened, since real-life stressors come in many different shapes and sizes. Conversely, perhaps it is not unreasonable to expect that individuals might be more readily engaged by some challenges than by others, and that, when we use different tasks in the laboratory, a person will react more to one task than to another. The implications of this hypothesis will be examined in Chapter 10 when discussing the Risk Identification Protocol.

As one last experimental example, consider some data from a study reported by Turner *et al.* (1990) in which 32 subjects completed four tasks, two speech tasks and two math tasks. Turner *et al.* (1990) presented heart rate and blood pressure data for all 32 subjects, showing considerable intertask consistency of reactivity scores. Here, however, data from only 23 subjects are presented. The reason for this is simple and deliberate. Hemodynamic data were also collected in that study, but these were available only for 23 of the 32 subjects. We shall presently explore the intertask consistency of the hemodynamic variables cardiac output and total peripheral resistance. Because it will prove informative to compare the intertask consistency of blood pressure reactivity with that of its underlying hemodynamic determinants, fairness demands that the hemodynamic data be compared with the data from precisely the same 23 subjects rather than all 32 subjects, even though the blood pressure data for this subsample look almost identical to those for the full sample of 32.

Table 5.4 presents the intertask consistency correlations for blood pressure reactivity.[2] Eleven of the 12 coefficients attained statistical significance. The coefficient magnitudes ranged from 0.39 to 0.80, with 11 of the 12 falling between 0.51 and 0.80. It may also be noted that, in all six cases, the systolic reactivity correlation for a particular task pairing was greater than the diastolic correlation. Thus, as for temporal stability, the evidence is greater for systolic reactivity than for diastolic reactivity. However, in the case of intertask consistency, diastolic values do not fall as far behind systolic (and heart rate) values as is the case for temporal stability.

[2]The verbalization speech task required subjects to read a passage high in informational content and then to describe aloud the substance of the article, while the interpersonal speech task required subjects to describe how they would act in the hypothetical situation of being refused permission to board an aircraft to travel to a very important and distant engagement. The serial subtraction math task required subjects to subtract 17 serially from a four-digit starting number, and the computer math task was a second-generation version of the interactive math task (MATH) described in Chapter 3.

Table 5.4. Intertask Correlations for Reactivity Scores
for Blood Pressure Variables (n = 23)

Variable	"Verbalization" speech	Serial subtraction	Computer math
Systolic blood pressure			
"Interpersonal" speech	0.73**	0.71**	0.77**
"Verbalization" speech		0.80**	0.65**
Serial subtraction			0.73**
Diastolic blood pressure			
"Interpersonal" speech	0.39	0.55**	0.71**
"Verbalization" speech		0.57**	0.51*
Serial subtraction			0.61**

*$p < 0.05$.
**$p < 0.01$.

Overall, these studies and others like them have provided a reasonable degree of evidence for intertask consistency of response to psychological stressors. It is probably true to say that the evidence for intertask consistency is not quite as compelling as that for temporal stability. However, various factors may cause our evaluations of intertask consistency to underestimate its true strength. Discussion of one of these follows.

Even though the two tasks being compared in intertask consistency investigations are usually completed in the same experimental session, separated by only a few minutes, they are not completed simultaneously. This sounds like a somewhat obvious statement—of course, only one task at a time is undertaken. However, it has a less obvious corollary. The fact that the two tasks are not completed contemporaneously means that any evaluation of intertask consistency also contains shades of temporal stability. Let us examine data from a couple of studies where, for various reasons, the exact same task was done twice within the same experimental session, the two occasions thus being very close in time.

First, as will be discussed further in Chapter 7, Carroll *et al.* (1985) reported a study in which subjects completed two bouts of a video game task within a single session. Heart rate reactivity scores for the two sessions were compared in what can be considered an evaluation of temporal stability across a very short time interval. Because the subjects in that study were twins, two correlations were actually computed, one for identical and one for nonidentical twins; coefficients of 0.75 and 0.77, respectively, were obtained. Second, Turner and Sherwood (1991) required subjects to complete two bouts of mental arithmetic in each of two postures, seated and standing, during the same experimental session. For systolic and diastolic pressure reactivity during the seated task, the test-retest correlations were 0.77 and 0.78, respectively; for values during the standing task the analogous coefficients were 0.63 and 0.74.

While these half dozen test-retest correlations came from different studies involving differing tasks and numbers of subjects, they are remarkably similar in magnitude. While finding the arithmetic average of correlation coefficients is not always to be recommended, we will do it here purely for the purpose of making a point. The mean of the six coefficients is 0.74. What does this tell us in the context of the investigation of intertask consistency? It tells us that even when *exactly the same task* is given on two occasions separated only by a few minutes, responses will not be identical; they will be similar, but not identical, as would be indicated by a coefficient of 1.00. Thus, when giving *two different tasks*, the best we can realistically expect is an intertask correlation of 0.74, *not* 1.00. That is, 0.74 is the ceiling of reasonable expectation.

As can be seen from Table 5.4 presented earlier, several of the coefficients approach this level. (Two of them actually exceed it; however, it is the point itself, not the precise value of 0.74, that is important here.) Thus, all things being considered, the support for the concept of intertask consistency of heart rate and blood pressure reactivity is reasonably strong.

Hemodynamic Variables

Sherwood, Dolan, and Light (1990b) examined the hemodynamic responses of 90 subjects to various tasks. While the different tasks gave rise to different patterns of hemodynamic responses, intertask correlations of blood pressure, cardiac output, and vascular resistance were significant in 39 of 40 comparisons made. The consistency of hemodynamic response patterning that these correlations suggested was then further explored by the *post hoc* formation of myocardial (or cardiac output) and vascular (or peripheral resistance) reactor groups, based on their responses to a competitive reaction time task. Thirty subjects whose blood pressure responses to this task were due to increased cardiac output were designated the high myocardial reactors, and 31 subjects whose blood pressure responses were associated with vascular resistance increases were designated the high vascular group. The contrasting pattern of hemodynamic responses displayed by these two reactivity groups was maintained across all the other stressors (including both active and passive tasks), suggesting that the hemodynamic basis of reactivity is an individual characteristic that is only partially modified by the coping demands of a specific situation.

The hemodynamic intertask stability shown by a subset of the subjects employed in the Turner *et al.* (1990) study has recently been examined. It was noted earlier, when presenting blood pressure data for this reduced sample, that the data now discussed could thus be directly compared with the data for blood pressure. Table 5.5 presents intertask correlations for cardiac output and total peripheral resistance reactivity scores. Eleven of 12 coefficients attained significance, and, of greater interest, the magnitudes of these 11 ranged from 0.49 to 0.90. These data can now be compared directly to the blood pressure data (see Table 5.4). It can be seen that the overall pattern and magnitudes of the coefficients for the hemodynamic variables are strikingly similar to those for blood pressure.

Finally here, intertask consistency of both blood pressure and hemodynamic variables has been assessed using the subject sample employed by Dr. Kathleen Light in a large-scale investigation of race and gender group influences on cardiovascular reactivity (see Light *et al.*,

Table 5.5. Intertask Correlations for Reactivity Scores for Hemodynamic Variables (n = 23)

Variable	"Verbalization" speech	Serial subtraction	Computer math
Cardiac output			
"Interpersonal" speech	0.78**	0.56**	0.52*
"Verbalization" speech		0.66**	0.63**
Serial subtraction			0.90**
Total peripheral resistance			
"Interpersonal" speech	0.69**	0.30	0.49*
"Verbalization" speech		0.52*	0.74**
Serial subtraction			0.81**

*$p < 0.05$.
**$p < 0.01$.

1993a). In a preliminary examination of a subset of this sample (36 subjects), intertask coefficients ranging from 0.37 to 0.75 were found for cardiac output responses, and coefficients ranging from 0.38 to 0.76 were found for peripheral resistance reactivity scores (see Turner *et al.*, 1991). More recently, similar correlations for intertask consistency based on the full sample of 128 of the subjects for whom complete hemodynamic data were available have been confirmed (Turner *et al.*, 1993b).

Evidence is thus accumulating that cardiac and vascular responses, the underlying determinants of blood pressure responses, show the same intertask consistency as do the blood pressure responses themselves. It would thus appear that the hemodynamic patterns underlying blood pressure responses are themselves reliable individual difference characteristics (Sherwood & Turner, 1992).

Discussion

Three attributes of individual differences in reactivity are of interest: temporal stability, intertask consistency, and laboratory-field generalizability. The first two of these have been examined in detail in this chapter (the third being discussed in Chapter 9).

The evidence for temporal stability of reactivity indicates a reasonable degree of stability for heart rate, blood pressure (at least systolic), and the hemodynamic variables of cardiac output and total peripheral resistance. This suggests that a given individual may be regarded as having a characteristic cardiovascular response predisposition when faced with a stressful situation. This stability adds very importantly to the evidence of individual differences obtained in single-test experiments; some of this evidence was presented at the start of this chapter. It appears that these differences are real, stable differences.

Demonstration of individual differences and their stability is a crucial prerequisite before considering the use of reactivity scores as a predictor of later disease. First, if everyone reacted in exactly the same way, reactivity would not be any help in predicting later disease, since not everyone develops cardiovascular pathology. Second, if people were to react very differently at different times, we would have no confidence in their reactivity score obtained in a single-session test. Reactivity may or may not turn out to be a good predictor, but this stability of individual differences makes it a legitimate candidate to be evaluated for predictive powers (see Chapter 10).

Evidence for intertask consistency of reactivity is also accumulating. As well as data for heart rate and blood pressure, recent data are now available for cardiac output and peripheral resistance. These data indicate that the hemodynamic patterns underlying blood pressure responses are themselves reliable individual difference characteristics. What this tells us is that individuals whose blood pressure responses are mediated primarily by peripheral resistance in one situation will tend to increase blood pressure in the same way in other situations. The same is also true for people who primarily mediate their blood pressure responses via cardiac influences. Interestingly, this level of hemodynamic consistency appears to be present even when the magnitudes of blood pressure responses in two situations are quite different. For example, a vascular reactor will tend to mediate both small and large blood pressure increases via increases in total peripheral resistance. The same principle applies for cardiac reactors. This observation provides further evidence that the use of hemodynamic variables in future research is likely to be highly informative.

In this chapter we have focused on the *individual factor*. While the *situational factor* is undoubtedly important, so too it seems is the individual one. We have seen evidence that considerable individual differences exist in cardiovascular responses to psychological stress, and that these differences show a reasonable degree of stability. While these differences alone *do not prove* hypothesized connections between reactivity and disease, they are *consistent with* observations from another aspect of stress research.

Levi (1974) discussed the diathesis-stress model of illness. This model, as do most current models of stress and illness, postulates that stress precipitates illness where there is an existing vulnerability, or *diathesis* (Carroll, 1992). In the diathesis-stress model, physiological predispositions toward a certain illness, psychosocial stimuli, and previously experienced environmental conditions will jointly determine many disease states (Gatchel *et al.*, 1989). Vulnerability can operate at a number of levels, including the biological, psychological, and social levels. While all are important, this chapter has focused on the biological factor in cardiovascular stress responses, and so we shall comment on only the biological level of vulnerability.

Some individuals may be predisposed to suffer disruption to specific biological systems in the face of stress (Carroll, 1992). Considerable individual differences in cardiovascular responses to stress have been documented in this chapter, and in due course Chapter 7 will present evidence that these individual differences reflect, at least in part, genetic predisposition. While it should be emphasized again that the present evidence alone is not conclusive, it may be the case that individual differences in cardiovascular stress responses reflect, to a certain degree, differences in predispositions to suffer from later cardiovascular disease.

Summary

Considerable individual differences exist in cardiovascular responses to psychological stress. Some individuals show large cardiovascular increases during a given task, while others show minimal alterations in cardiovascular activity. These differences are not related to how engaging individuals find the task, nor to how well they do on the task.

There is now reasonable evidence of temporal stability of cardiovascular stress responses. If an individual reacts highly to a given task on one occasion, it is likely that he or she will react similarly when the same task is completed on another occasion. There is also evidence of intertask consistency of response, particularly for hemodynamic variables. If an individual mediates blood pressure responses during a task primarily via one hemodynamic route, it is likely that he or she will do the same during a different task, even if the magnitude of the blood pressure response is different during the two tasks. It therefore appears that an individual's biological program may be primed for a predetermined level, and mode, of response in the face of psychological stress.

Further Reading

1. Kasprowicz, A.L., Manuck, S.B., Malkoff, S.B., & Krantz, D.S. (1990). Individual differences in behaviorally evoked cardiovascular response: Temporal stability and hemodynamic patterning. *Psychophysiology, 27,* 605–619.

2. Llabre, M.M., Saab, P.G., Hurwitz, B.E., Schneiderman, N., Frame, C.A., Spitzer, S., & Phillips, D. (1993). The stability of cardiovascular parameters under different behavioral challenges: One-year follow-up. *International Journal of Psychophysiology, 14,* 241–248.

3. McKinney, M.E., Miner, M.H., Ruddel, H., McIlvain, H.E., Witte, H., Buell, J.C., Eliot, R.S., & Grant, L.B. (1985). The standardized mental stress test protocol: Test-retest reliability and comparison with ambulatory blood pressure monitoring. *Psychophysiology, 22,* 453–463.

4. Manuck, S.B., & Garland, F.N. (1980). Stability of individual differences in cardio-vascular reactivity: A thirteen-month follow-up. *Physiology and Behavior, 24,* 621–624.
5. Manuck, S.B., Kasprowicz, A.L., Monroe, S.M., Larkin, K.T., & Kaplan, J.R. (1989). Psychophysiological reactivity as a dimension of individual differences. In N. Schneiderman, S.M. Weiss, & P.G. Kaufmann (Eds.), *Handbook of research methods in cardiovascular behavioral medicine* (pp. 365–382). New York: Plenum.
6. Sherwood, A., Dolan, C.A., & Light, K.C. (1990). Hemodynamics of blood pressure responses during active and passive coping. *Psychophysiology, 37,* 656–668.
7. Sherwood, A., Turner, J.R., Light, K.C., & Blumenthal, J.A. (1990). Temporal stability of the hemodynamics of cardiovascular reactivity. *International Journal of Psychophysiology, 10,* 95–98.
8. Steptoe, A., & Vögele, C. (1991). Methodology of mental stress testing in cardiovascular research. *Circulation, 83,* (Suppl. II), II-14–II-24.
9. Turner, J.R. (1989). Individual differences in heart rate response during behavioral challenge. *Psychophysiology, 26,* 497–505.
10. Turner, J.R., Sherwood, A., & Light, K.C. (1992). *Individual differences in cardiovascular response to stress.* New York: Plenum.

CHAPTER 6

Cardiac-Metabolic Dissociation: Additional Heart Rates during Psychological Stress

The main focus of this chapter is on basic experimental research conducted to demonstrate that the large cardiac increases displayed by certain individuals during psychological stress are indeed over and above the adjustments dictated by the physical, or metabolic, demands of the situation. However, in addition to examining this cardiac-metabolic dissociation, the chapter provides a good opportunity to illustrate several of the points discussed in earlier chapters with examples from actual experiments. Some of the tasks discussed earlier, the basic psychophysiological strategy of investigating reactivity, and the phenomenon of individual differences in psychophysiological response to psychological challenge will all be encountered here.

Physiological responses to stress have been suggested as a possible contributor to cardiovascular pathology. While several cardiovascular parameters are of importance in this line of research, the present chapter concentrates exclusively on the quantification of heart rate change in response to psychological stress. While a common and recommended way of representing such change is to subtract a baseline value from the task level, thus yielding a reactivity score, this chapter discusses "additional heart rate" as an alternative.

The heart rate increases seen in response to laboratory psychological stressors appear to be metabolically excessive, for the tasks are specifically designed with response requirements that demand minimal physical activity. This uncoupling of cardiac and metabolic processes is of great interest in itself, since it represents a breakdown of their orderly relationship. In addition, as we have seen in previous chapters, such metabolically inappropriate responses have been discussed in relation to hypertension. Two possibilities are of interest. First, such responses may play a role in the pathogenesis of hypertension (Obrist, 1981). Second, while not being causally related, they may be early indicators of the later development of hypertension (Manuck & Krantz, 1986). The present chapter does not attempt to address these issues directly, but adopts the standpoint that, since such cardiac responses are of interest, it might be useful to explore alternative methods of their quantification.

Additional Heart Rate: The First Studies

An intimate and biologically sensible relationship exists between cardiac and somatic processes. The heart is a supreme example of biomechanical engineering, and, under normal circumstances, it operates with elegant economy. As striate muscle activity increases, so too does cardiac activity, thereby providing muscles with the extra oxygen required. During recent years, however, it has become apparent that under certain conditions this cardiac-somatic link breaks down, and increases in cardiac activity appear in the absence of parallel elevations in somatic activity. This phenomenon is called *cardiac-metabolic dissociation.*

Early Studies

In 1974, Blix, Stromme, and Ursin reported an examination of the relationship between cardiovascular activity and oxygen consumption in helicopter and transport aircraft pilots engaged in flying maneuvers. Physiological parameters were measured in two contexts: (1) during flight operations, comprising a 10-minute demanding training program for the helicopter pilots, and actual scheduled operations, including take-off and landing, for the transport carrier pilots; and (2) a rest period and maximal work on a treadmill. Heart rate was obtained telemetrically, and oxygen consumption determined by subsequent analysis of expired air collected in Douglas bags.

Physiological values obtained during rest and maximal exercise were used to construct plots of heart rate against oxygen consumption, it being assumed that under steady-state or aerobic exercise there exists a linear relationship between these two parameters. Oxygen consumption during the flight operations was then used in conjunction with the regression plots to determine expected, or predicted, heart rate; the difference between this value and the recorded one was termed the "additional heart rate" (Blix et al., 1974).

Actual heart rates were considerably greater than the values predicted from contemporary oxygen consumption values, the average additional heart rate being 23.8 bpm. The authors concluded that additional heart rate "is a reliable and valid indicator of psychological activation which goes beyond somatomotor activations."

In a later study, Stromme, Wikeby, Blix, and Ursin (1978) tested 13 parachute trainees at the Norwegian Army Parachute Training School. A similar but more sophisticated methodology for calculating additional heart rate was employed. On this occasion the regression plots for heart rate and oxygen consumption were more rigorously constructed from measurements taken during rest and three moderate workloads on a bicycle ergometer. During the jump training, heart rate and oxygen consumption were recorded as in the Blix et al. (1974) study. Just before and just after actual jumps from the training tower, average additional heart rate values of 40 bpm and 60 bpm, respectively, were observed.

Figure 6.1 represents diagrammatically the calculation of an additional heart rate value for a single subject. In this example, rest and four workloads have been used to generate five heart rate/oxygen consumption data points. A regression plot has been calculated and drawn using these points. Also shown is a heart rate/oxygen consumption data point obtained during a psychological task. Use of the actual oxygen consumption and the regression line enables calculation of the predicted heart rate. The difference between this value and the actual heart rate is thus designated the "additional heart rate."

Laboratory Investigation Using Nonhuman Subjects

The next phase of the examination of this topic moves into the psychophysiological laboratory. While nonlaboratory, or "real-world" investigations are of great importance, controllable laboratory representations of behavioral stress are also very valuable since they offer the control necessary for the experimental manipulation of parameters of

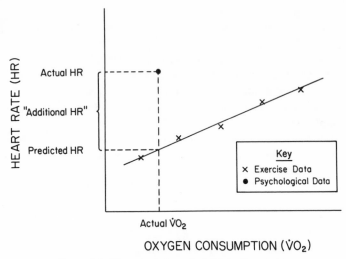

Figure 6.1. The calculation of additional heart rate.

interest. Two laboratory studies using nonhuman subjects are particularly noteworthy.

Langer, Obrist, and McCubbin (1979) examined this issue using
dogs. The implantation of aortic electromagnetic flow probes facilitated
measurement of cardiac output, while implantation of catheters in the
right ventricle and aorta enabled the arterial-mixed venous oxygen
content difference to be calculated; knowledge of cardiac output per-
mits the latter value to be converted to a measure of oxygen uptake. The
animals participated in two tasks: exercise on a treadmill, and a sig-
naled shock-avoidance task. The exercise task comprised three grades
of exercise, designated as light, intermediate, and heavy. This permitted, for each dog, the plotting of cardiac output against arterial-mixed
venous oxygen content difference; the line of best fit and the 95%
prediction interval representing this relationship during exercise was
thus drawn (see Figure 1, p. 228, in Langer *et al.*, 1979).

Of the six animals exposed to these procedures, four displayed
clear evidence of a metabolically exaggerated cardiac increase during
shock avoidance; significantly less oxygen was extracted during avoidance than during exercise at comparable levels of cardiac output. The
authors interpreted their results as evidence of "overperfusion of sys-

temic circulation," since cardiac output appeared "relatively excessive for any given level of blood oxygen extraction during shock avoidance" (Langer *et al.*, 1979, p. H228).

In the study reported by Sherwood, Brener, and Moncur (1983), heart rate and oxygen consumption were measured in rats during behavioral adaptation to an avoidance conditioning task. The metabolic relevance of heart rate responses during the stressor was evaluated on the basis of regression equations fitted to habituation data for each individual animal. Interest focused on the hypothesis that environmental conditions requiring high levels of motor preparation may induce greater "suprametabolic elevations" in heart rate than conditions similar in all respects except the level of motor readiness demanded (Sherwood *et al.*, 1983).

Twelve rats were divided into two equal groups, matched for weight and age. Animals in the high predictability group were tested under conditions where the onset of each imperative stimulus occurred at a fixed interval of 5 seconds following the onset of each discriminative stimulus. In the low predictability condition, imperative stimuli occurred at random intervals following the onset of the discriminative stimuli.

In both conditions, shock avoidance required a brief, rapid-running response during the imperative stimulus. The crucial difference between high and low predictability conditions, therefore, was that the times at which this avoidance response would be required were highly uncertain for the low predictability group; the converse was true for the high predictability group.

The hypothesis that this experimental manipulation would lead to additional heart rates being displayed more of the time by low predictability subjects, since they would need to maintain a higher level of motor readiness than high predictability subjects, was supported by the results. While oxygen consumption and ambulation did not differ between groups, heart rates were significantly higher for the low predictability group. When average group additional heart rates were computed—on the basis of concurrent oxygen consumption and the heart rate/oxygen consumption regressions obtained during habituation—for each of two 3-hour conditioning sessions, the low predictability group displayed significantly and dramatically higher values, which also significantly increased over the duration of the sessions.

Further evidence of metabolically excessive cardiac adjustments is provided by this report. In addition, the influence of uncertainty is highlighted. This factor has come to be widely regarded as important in determining situations that may evoke suprametabolic activity in human subjects.

Laboratory Assessment of Suprametabolic Cardiac Activity in Humans

The laboratory investigation of metabolically excessive cardiac activity during active psychological stressors has been guided by the elegant series of experiments conducted by Obrist, Langer, Sherwood, and colleagues. Early studies (see Obrist *et al.*, 1974; Obrist *et al.*, 1978) reported heart rate levels that appeared excessive relative to task somatic demands. Sampling of concurrent oxygen consumption facilitated more direct appraisal of the metabolic relevance of observed cardiac changes (Gliner *et al.*, 1982). More recently, the advent of highly sophisticated systems, such as that developed by Langer *et al.* (1985) and that described by Turner *et al.* (1983), has permitted the continuous assessment of oxygen consumption during laboratory experimentation using human subjects (see Langer *et al.*, 1985).

Present methodology has evolved to comprise continuous measurement of cardiac and metabolic parameters during both psychological and physical stressors, and compelling evidence of behaviorally induced violations of the heart's biologically sensible economy of action has been documented. It is this evidence that is now discussed.

Additional Heart Rate during Laboratory Stressors

Turner and Carroll (1985a) conducted a study in which 20 subjects undertook two active psychological stressors, a video game and a mental arithmetic task, and completed a graded isotonic exercise task on an exercise bicycle. Heart rate was recorded on a Beckman Dynograph, and metabolic and respiratory activity were monitored using a Beckman Metabolic Cart (see Turner *et al.*, 1983). Of the range of metabolic and respiratory variables measured, we shall focus only on oxygen consumption.

The mean values for heart rate and oxygen consumption for each of the nine measurement periods in this study are presented in Table 6.1. To calculate additional heart rates during the psychological stressors, it was necessary to construct regressions for each subject separately.

Table 6.1. Mean Heart Rate and Oxygen Consumption
Values for All Measurement Periods

Measurement period	Heart rate (bpm)	Oxygen consumption (mlpm)[a]
Video game		
Baseline	75.1	244.5
Task	85.4	374.0
Mental arithmetic task		
Baseline	74.0	249.5
Task	85.7	294.0
Exercise bicycle		
Rest	73.5	306.0
Level 1	90.4	679.5
Level 2	98.3	934.5
Level 3	110.6	1204.0
Level 4	126.0	1531.5

Adapted from Turner & Carroll, 1985a.
[a]Milliliters per minute.

Consequently, physiological values during the exercise task were used to obtain individual regressions of heart rate on oxygen consumption. Figure 6.2 presents examples of these regressions for four subjects (the dotted lines represent 95% confidence limits for the regressions). In addition to the regression lines constructed from the exercise data, data points for the psychological stressors are shown, along with data points for their respective baselines. These four examples are presented because they illustrate the range of profiles evident during these stressors. Two subjects were particularly reactive to one of the two tasks, one subject was quite reactive to them both, and one subject showed virtually no heart rate increase during either task.

These regression equations were then used in conjunction with actual oxygen consumption values during mental arithmetic and the video game and their respective baseline periods to compute "predicted heart rate values." These predicted heart rate values were then subtracted from heart rate values actually recorded to obtain additional heart rate values. The mean additional heart rate values were +12.6 bpm and +2.7 bpm for mental arithmetic task and baseline periods, respectively, and +9.0 bpm and +3.8 bpm for video game task and baseline periods, respectively. The means, however, conceal enormous individ-

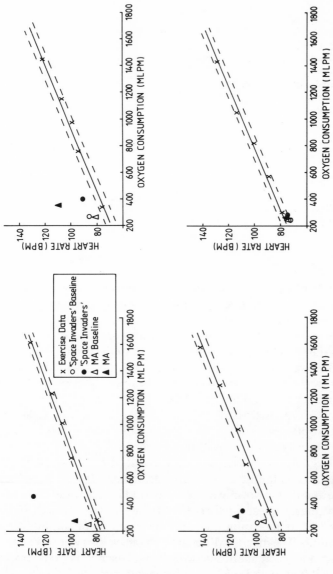

Figure 6.2. Heart rate and oxygen consumption for four individual subjects during isotonic exercise and during the psychological challenges and their respective baselines. Also shown are regression lines for the exercise data. Reprinted with permission from Turner & Carroll, 1985. ©The Society for Psychophysiological Research.

ual variation; for the mental arithmetic task period, values ranged from −3.6 bpm to +34.7 bpm, and for the video game from −4.9 bpm to +42.6 bpm.

The number of errors made during mental arithmetic and three performance scores for the video game (first score, best score, and improvement, defined as the difference between first and best score) were then correlated with the appropriate additional heart rate values to examine the possible influence of performance; none of the correlations obtained even approached the magnitude necessary for statistical significance. Finally, self-report of mental engagement during the task periods was examined and was found to be similarly unrelated to additional heart rate.

Actual heart rates during the two psychological stressors employed in this study, then, were substantially greater for the vast majority of subjects than the heart rates predicted from concurrent metabolic demand and heart rate/oxygen consumption regression equations generated by the graded isotonic exercise task. Tasks that are psychologically challenging but pose only minimal physical demands can therefore elicit heart rate reactions in certain individuals that are additional to the adjustments predicted on the basis of energy expenditure. The enormous individual variation evident should be emphasized, as should the independence of additional heart rate from both performance and perceived engagement in the tasks.

Several other informative points arise from this study. First, the pretask baselines themselves were characterized by small additional heart rates. Instead of inducing true resting states, these periods gave rise to anticipatorily mediated heart rate elevations. This result supports Obrist and Light's (1988) contention that cardiovascular measures taken immediately before a stressor may be inappropriate for baseline purposes. The more traditional representation of heart rate change in such circumstances is heart rate reactivity, defined as "task heart rate minus baseline heart rate." Thus, if an immediately pretask baseline is used, the elevated nature of the baseline may give rise to underestimation of the increase from true resting level to task heart rate level. The use of additional heart rate as the index of heart rate change circumvents this problem.

Second, additional heart rate takes into account the differing metabolic demands of the physical response requirements of different tasks. Both tasks in this study were chosen because they had "minimal" physical demand. However, the video game task required (or at least elicited) more muscular activity than initially intended. This may have been due to the use of arm and shoulder musculature, to a small extent, and to "extra vigorous" pressing of control keys. The initial analysis for oxygen consumption revealed that, while the metabolic demands of both tasks were (intentionally) very small in absolute terms, the video game task required significantly more energy expenditure than did mental arithmetic. A larger part of the increase in heart rate from resting to task levels was therefore due to metabolically *appropriate* responses for the video game than for mental arithmetic. The additional heart rate methodology has the advantage (compared with heart rate reactivity scores) that it takes into account the differences in oxygen consumption demand of each task's response requirements, and also any incidental physical activity on the part of subjects eliciting metabolically justified heart rate increases that might otherwise appear unwarranted.

Although these arguments are true, it should be emphasized that, for many practical purposes, heart rate reactivity scores do provide a good indication of a person's responsiveness. If an individual yields an additional heart rate score of $+40$ bpm and a heart rate reactivity score of $+34.7$ bpm—the difference being due to the reasons described above—it is safe to assume that, had the heart rate reactivity score only been obtained, this individual would be correctly classified as a "high reactor." Because no absolute heart rate change value delineates high from low reactors, the small differences may not be crucial. In other words, this work demonstrates that if a person shows a large heart rate reactivity score during one of our psychological stressors, it is extremely likely that this heart rate response is metabolically excessive.

In this study, heart rate reactivity scores were also calculated. They were significantly correlated with additional heart rate scores; $r(18) = 0.91$, $p < .01$ for mental arithmetic, and $r(18) = 0.83$, $p < .01$ for the video game. While both correlations are high, the extra 14% of explained variance in the case of mental arithmetic is probably a direct result of the lower energy expenditure demands of that task's response requirements.

Choice of the Comparator Exercise Task

Carroll, Turner, and Rogers (1987) used a graded static, or isometric, exercise task instead of the dynamic, or isotonic, exercise task (the bicycle task) employed by Turner and Carroll (1985a). This task consisted of subjects sitting in a chair and holding their leg at three successive heights above the floor. While this task produced steeper heart rate/oxygen consumption regression slopes than did dynamic exercise on the bicycle ergometer, additional heart rates during mental arithmetic and the video game were still evident, even though their values were smaller. However, Carroll *et al.* (1987) argued that dynamic exercise remained the proper choice in studies using heart rate as the measure of cardiac performance, since cardiac output, the real parameter of interest (see the final section in this chapter), is probably reflected reliably by heart rate during both dynamic exercise (Wilmore & Norton, 1975) and active psychological challenge (Sherwood *et al.*, 1986), but not during graded static exercise (Bezucha *et al.*, 1982).

A second study examined the issue of whether upper body or lower body dynamic exercise might be more appropriate as the comparator exercise task against which to judge the metabolic appropriateness of heart rate adjustments during psychological challenge. Turner *et al.* (1988b) incorporated both upper and lower body dynamic exercise tasks in a within-subject design employing 22 subjects to facilitate their direct comparison in this context. The regression lines generated by the two tasks were extremely similar. Additional heart rates were then calculated separately for each comparator task. Rigorous analysis of variance revealed no significant differences whatsoever between the values calculated using the two tasks. This similarity is captured succinctly in the two correlation coefficients that were subsequently calculated between the two sets of additional heart rates; for mental arithmetic, $r(20) = 0.93$ $(p < .01)$, and for the video game, $r(20) = 0.87$ $(p < .01)$. While the hemodynamic effects of upper body and lower body exercise may vary somewhat, they yielded almost identical heart rate/oxygen consumption regression equations and, accordingly, generated strikingly similar additional heart rates.

From a theoretical perspective, either upper or lower body exercise could serve equally well in this capacity. However, practical considerations support the candidacy of the bicycle ergometer task. This task is much simpler to explain to subjects and, subjectively, it feels much more "natural." The task can be completed easily and without any concerns on the part of the subject. These studies provide some experimental support for the intrinsically appealing choice of the bicycle ergometer as the exercise best-suited comparator task.

Effects of Level of Task Difficulty

Obrist *et al.* (1978) reported an experiment where the subjects' success in a shock-avoidance task was manipulated by altering task difficulty. There were three conditions: easy, reasonably difficult, and impossible. It was hypothesized that little cardiac reactivity would occur in the easy and impossible conditions, for in both conditions the subjects would not be actively involved in struggling to cope. The easy condition is dealt with quite readily, while subjects in the impossible condition would cease trying after a few trials as they realized the nature of the task. On the other hand, it was hypothesized that the difficult condition, in which subjects could cope fairly successfully as long as they continued to try hard, was expected to result in the largest sustained cardiac increases.

Results showed that, although initial average heart rate increases for all three conditions were nearly 20 bpm above baseline, after 14 minutes the average heart rate in the easy and impossible conditions had fallen to 3 bpm and 5 bpm above baseline, respectively, whereas in the reasonably difficult condition average heart rate had fallen only to 10 bpm above baseline. While these findings are indicative that the difficult condition led to the greatest metabolically inappropriate adjustments, the lack of continuous metabolic assessment precludes unequivocal assertions. Accordingly, two studies were performed to explore the effect of task difficulty on additional heart rate.

In the first study (Carroll *et al.*, 1986a), mental arithmetic and a Raven's Matrices task were used. These tasks lent themselves easily to difficulty manipulation, and it was possible to keep motor demands constant across difficulty levels. For each task, three levels of difficulty were selected; these were termed easy, hard and impossible. For mental arithmetic, pilot work, using students from the same population from which the subject sample was drawn, revealed that the easy problems were indeed handled easily. The hard problems were selected from those used previously by Turner and Carroll (1985a). Problems in the impossible category, consisting of multiplication and division of two 2-digit or 3-digit numbers, were not actually "impossible" to solve, but they were judged to be so in the time available for each trial.

For Raven's Matrices, easy and hard problems consisted of sets A and B, and sets D and E, respectively, of Raven's Standard Progressive Matrices (Raven, 1960); the impossible problems comprised examples 13 to 36 of Raven's Advanced Progressive Matrices (Raven, 1962). The matrices were reproduced as slides and presented to subjects by means of a slide viewer. It should again be noted that the impossible problems were not actually "impossible" to solve, but on the basis of a pilot study they were judged to be so in the available trial time.

For mental arithmetic, mean additional heart rates during the easy, hard, and impossible conditions were 3.8 bpm, 7.8 bpm, and 7.4 bpm, respectively; for Raven's Matrices, the respective values were 4.6 bpm, 7.1 bpm, and 7.0 bpm. Analysis of variance and subsequent *post hoc* comparison indicated that, for both tasks, additional heart rates were less during the easy condition than during either the hard or the impossible condition ($p < .01$), but that the values during the hard and impossible conditions did not differ significantly from each other.

Results obtained were somewhat different from initial expectations. The results of Obrist *et al.* (1978) had led to the expectation that relatively little cardiac activity would be seen during the easy and impossible conditions. These expectations were only partially fulfilled, since the impossible condition continued to elicit equally sizable cardiac reactions as did the hard condition. In speculating as to why the impossible condition led to this continued cardiac activity, one possibility immediately suggested itself. It may be that insufficient time was allowed and that, with a longer experience of impossibility, subjects would have become disengaged from the task, and that this disengagement would then have led to lower responses. A second study was undertaken to evaluate this hypothesis.

Carroll, Turner, and Prasad (1986b) described what in essence was an attempt to replicate the previous finding that additional heart rates are sensitive to differences in task difficulty. The key difference was that on this occasion just one psychological stressor—mental arithmetic—was employed in which the blocks of trials corresponding to the three levels of difficulty lasted *twice as long* as in the previous study. On this occasion, difficulty level exerted an unambiguous effect on additional heart rate. Both the easy and the impossible conditions elicited significantly less additional heart rate than did the hard condition. The mean values were 4.2 bpm, 8.0 bpm, and 5.3 bpm for the easy, hard, and impossible conditions, respectively. These results were very much in line with those of Obrist *et al.* (1978), since the greatest mean cardiac response was seen at the hard level as opposed to the easy and impossible conditions.

These studies show that, in order for an individual's characteristic cardiac response under stress to be seen, that individual must be given a task that is neither too easy nor too hard. A task of appropriate difficulty will best engage the subject psychologically and therefore lead to that individual's characteristic level of cardiac response under stress being seen. The studies provide experimental support for the rationale behind tasks employing standardized flexibility (seen in Chapter 3).

Additional Heart Rates and Heart Rate Reactivity Scores

The correlations between additional heart rates and heart rate reactivity scores reported earlier in this chapter merit further discussion. The highly significant relationships suggest powerfully that heart rate reactivity scores provide a very good approximation of additional heart rates in the type of situations with which we are concerned—that is, experimental tasks designed specifically to be low in physical demand (and hence metabolic demand). Although it is true that the additional heart rate methodology explicitly captures the extent to which heart rate responses are metabolically excessive—a quality that makes the methodology very useful in precise theoretical formulations concerning such cardiac events (see Turner, 1988)—these correlations show that in most cases the use of heart rate reactivity scores is perfectly acceptable.

In addition, the calculation of reactivity scores does not require individuals to be subjected to the rigorous regime necessary to represent cardiac changes in terms of additional heart rate (i.e., continuous metabolic assessment and the completion of an exercise task in addition to the psychological tasks). The calculation of simple reactivity scores, calculated as the arithmetic difference between task level and baseline level, therefore seems a very useful index of cardiac change. Indeed, throughout this book the vast majority of research discussed represents change in heart rate in terms of such reactivity scores.

Additional Cardiac Output

At this point, one implicit assumption of these additional heart rate studies must be dealt with. In terms of its relevance to potential disease, which is a central theme of this text, heart rate is taken as an implicit index of cardiac output in these studies. It is actually metabolically excessive increases in cardiac output, not heart rate per se, that are hypothesized to play a role in disease development. As we know from Chapter 2, cardiac output is the product of heart rate and stroke volume. It is therefore mathematically possible for an increase in heart rate to be associated with a *decrease* in cardiac output; all that is needed for this to happen is the appropriate decrease in stroke volume. However, studies that have evaluated stroke volume changes during psychological challenge have shown that this large decrease is not seen; stroke volume shows little change in these circumstances (e.g., Sherwood *et al.*, 1986). This evidence strongly suggests that the heart rate increases seen in these additional heart rate experiments would have occurred in conjunction with minimally altered stroke volumes, leading to metabolically excessive cardiac outputs. However, it must be stated explicitly at this point that we must remain aware of this limitation of the additional heart rate strategy.

This limitation was circumvented in the studies discussed next. Sherwood *et al.* (1986) reported a study in which the technique of impedance cardiography was employed to measure cardiac output itself. Cardiac output and oxygen consumption were monitored while subjects completed a graded exercise task on a bicycle ergometer and a reaction time task. On this occasion, regression lines describing the cardiac output/oxygen consumption relationship during exercise were obtained for each subject individually. For the group as a whole, cardiac output was elevated during the reaction time task with respect to baseline and was comparable to the levels observed with a light exercise load. In contrast, oxygen consumption did not change significantly. Convincing evidence of metabolically exaggerated cardiac output during behavioral challenge was thus provided.

Moreover, Carroll and colleagues have reported evidence demonstrating that, just as for heart rate, some individuals show evidence of considerable additional cardiac output when faced with psychological stress (Carroll *et al.*, 1990; Carroll *et al.*, 1991). Finally, van Doornen's group has also provided similar evidence (e.g., van Doornen & de Geus, 1989).

These studies represent the culmination of a whole line of investigation designed to look for evidence of metabolically inappropriate cardiac output in human subjects during psychological stress. Oxygen consumption is not frequently measured for these purposes in behavioral medicine experiments now (although it certainly is for other purposes such as determination of aerobic fitness levels, a topic dis-

cussed in Chapter 8). The experimental protocol required for the determination of suprametabolic adjustments is rigorous, and it means that
subjects are unable to talk to experimenters because of the breathing
equipment they must wear. Most studies in this field, therefore, now
operate under the implicit assumption that large cardiovascular adjustments seen during the studies will be metabolically inappropriate; these
studies choose tasks with minimal physical demands. The results
reviewed in this chapter provide solid evidence for the validity of this
assumption. Indeed, the categorization of large cardiac responses during psychological stress as suprametabolic has become axiomatic.

Summary

During psychological stress, some individuals display cardiac adjustments that are in excess of concurrent metabolic demand. These
responses are called *suprametabolic*. One strategy that has been used to
demonstrate this is the *additional heart rate* methodology. In addition to
measuring heart rate during the stressor, oxygen consumption (an
index of metabolic demand) is measured, and subjects also complete a
dynamic (isotonic) exercise task. For each individual subject, the relationship between heart rate and oxygen consumption during exercise is
used as a comparator against which to judge heart rate increases during
the psychological stressors. During these stressors, some individuals
show heart rates much higher than would be expected on the basis of
concurrent metabolic demand. The difference between metabolically
expected heart rate and actual heart rate is called additional heart rate.
A considerable range of individual differences exists between subjects
in these values.

Additional heart rate scores and heart rate reactivity scores are
highly correlated during the type of stressors used in current cardiovascular behavioral medicine research (i.e., tasks that have been deliberately designed to be minimally physically demanding). This means
that heart rate reactivity scores, which are much easier to obtain, are a
useful and practical way of quantifying metabolically excessive cardiac
changes during psychological stress.

Studies that have measured cardiac output along with oxygen
consumption show that metabolically excessive cardiac output itself
occurs in certain individuals during stress. They also suggest that, if

only heart rate is measured during these types of tasks, additional heart rate is a reasonable index of additional cardiac output.

Further Reading

1. Blix, A.S., Stromme, S.B., & Ursin, H. (1974). Additional heart rate—An indicator of psychological activation. *Aerospace Medicine, 45*, 1219–1222.
2. Carroll, D., Turner, J.R., & Prasad, R. (1986). The effects of level of difficulty of mental arithmetic challenge on heart rate and oxygen consumption. *International Journal of Psychophysiology, 4*, 167–173.
3. Langer, A.W., McCubbin, J.A., Stoney, C.M., Hutcheson, J.S., Charlton, J.D., & Obrist, P.A. (1985). Cardiopulmonary adjustments during exercise and an aversive reaction time task: Effects of beta-adrenoceptor blockade. *Psychophysiology, 22*, 59–68.
4. Langer, A.W., Obrist, P.A., & McCubbin, J.A. (1979). Hemodynamic and metabolic adjustments during exercise and shock avoidance in dogs. *American Journal of Physiology, 5*, H225–H230.
5. Sherwood, A., Allen, M.T., Obrist, P.A., & Langer, A.W. (1986). Evaluation of beta-adrenergic influences on cardiovascular and metabolic adjustments to physical and psychological stress. *Psychophysiology, 23*, 89–104.
6. Sherwood, A., Brener, J., & Moncur, D. (1983). Information and states of motor readiness: Their effects on the covariation of heart rate and energy expenditure. *Psychophysiology, 20*, 513–529.
7. Stoney, C.M., Langer, A.W., & Gelling, P.D. (1986). The effects of menstrual cycle phase on cardiovascular and pulmonary responses to physical and psychological stress. *Psychophysiology, 23*, 393–402.
8. Stromme, S.B., Wikeby, P.C., Blix, A.S., & Ursin, H. (1978). Additional heart rate. In H. Ursin, E. Baade, & S. Levine (Eds.), *Psychobiology of stress* (pp. 83–89). London: Academic Press.
9. Turner, J.R., & Carroll, D. (1985). Heart rate and oxygen consumption during mental arithmetic, a video game, and graded exercise: Further evidence of metabolically-exaggerated cardiac adjustments? *Psychophysiology, 22*, 261–267.
10. van Doornen, L.J.P., & de Geus, E.J.C. (1989). Aerobic fitness and the cardiovascular response to stress. *Psychophysiology, 26*, 17–28.

CHAPTER 7

Genetic Determinants of Individual Differences in Cardiovascular Reactivity

In this chapter we shall explore the genetic origins of individual differences in cardiovascular reactivity by examining studies that have employed the classical twin design to investigate the genetic and environmental determination of individual variation in cardiovascular response to psychological challenge. While the following research provides a good example of how behavior genetics can usefully be employed in behavioral medicine, it is not the only case of the successful marriage of these two disciplines. Other instances include the study of metabolic rate (Hewitt *et al.*, 1991), obesity (Fabsitz *et al.*, 1992; Stunkard *et al.*, 1986; see also Stunkard, 1991), type A behavior (Sims *et al.*, 1991; Tambs *et al.*, 1992), and addictive behaviors including smoking (Carmelli *et al.*, 1992) and drinking (Heath *et al.*, 1991). The interfacing of behavior genetic analysis strategies and behavioral medicine experimental paradigms is likely to increase in the future as the power of these genetic strategies is realized more and more by researchers in behavioral medicine (see Turner *et al.*, 1993a).

Before proceeding to look at twin studies of cardiovascular reactivity, it is of interest to see what bodies of evidence suggested that twin studies might be informative. We have already seen the evidence suggesting that several psychological stressors elicit metabolically excessive cardiac reactivity in certain individuals (Chapter 6), and we have noted the observed stability of individual differences in cardiovascular reactivity in such circumstances (Chapter 5). Two other relevant lines of inquiry concern the familial aggregation of blood pressure, and the relationship between subjects' cardiovascular reactivity and their parents' blood pressure status. We shall look at these in turn.

Familial Aggregation of Blood Pressure

Many authors (e.g., Feinleib, 1979; Feinleib *et al.*, 1975; Kannel, 1979; Klein, 1979) have acknowledged the importance of genetic factors in determining blood pressure levels, and Pickering (1968) concluded that between 33% and 64% of the variance in blood pressure is the result of hereditary factors.

It must be remembered, however, that it is difficult to separate genetic and environmental effects in a human population unambiguously. As Kannel (1979) noted: "Hypertension is indeed a family matter, but this does not necessarily reflect only genetic influences" (p. 54). A major problem is the fact that "the closer individuals are genetically, the more similar their environments are likely to be" (Feinleib, 1979, p. 46). An awareness of the interaction between genetic influences and environmental factors is also essential. While genetic factors "undoubtedly affect individual susceptibility to nongenetic promoters of cardiovascular disease," (Kannel, 1979, p. 49), in turn this predisposition may be either "muted or enhanced by environmental influences" (Kannel, 1979, p. 55).

Support for the involvement of genetic factors in familial blood pressure aggregation came from the Framingham Heart Study (see Kannel & Sorlie, 1979). This was a prospective cardiovascular study of 5,209 men and women; initial examinations were followed by eight biennial examinations. For example, one result from this study concerned 609 pairs of siblings aged between 30 and 60 years on initial examination. Blood pressure correlations between siblings evident on initial examination remained essentially constant over successive subsequent examinations despite the fact that the individuals largely lived apart during the 16-year period of the study (Feinleib, 1979). There is also evidence that shared environmental factors alone cannot account for familial variation in blood pressure. Similar longitudinal study of the relationship of blood pressure in spouses living together revealed no tendency for correlations between them to increase over time. Thus, "sharing a common environment, eating at a common table, and sharing common life problems" would not seem to enhance the correlations between blood pressure levels of spouses (Feinleib, 1979, p. 40). Taken together, these findings suggest the importance of genetic factors in familial aggregation of blood pressure, but they do not confirm it since both findings might be interpreted as suggesting that all of the damage is done by the family environment prior to adulthood.

In addition to the family studies mentioned, genetic involvement in hypertension is further indicated by the results of cross-breeding studies with rats and by research using human twins as subjects. Lawler and colleagues have reported a series of interesting experiments, which initially focused on the Spontaneously Hypertensive Rat, a genetic strain especially susceptible to hypertension. Lawler *et al.* (1980) argued that this was not a particularly helpful model for studying the effects of psychological stress since the animal's genetics are such that eventual development of hypertension is almost certain, regardless of the presence of stress. Lawler *et al.* (1980) thus cross-bred the Spontaneously Hypertensive Rat with normotensive control animals (the Wistar-Kyoto strain). The resulting strain developed systolic pressures in the borderline hypertensive range, and was thus called the Borderline Hypertensive Rat. An experimental group was then subjected to a shock-avoidance conflict paradigm. At the end of 12 weeks these animals had developed systolic levels approaching 190 mmHg, while a control group's levels had remained about 150 mmHg. Thus, the Borderline Hypertensive Rat became severely hypertensive only when exposed to psychological stress.

Lawler, Barker, Hubbard, and Schaub (1981) substantiated this finding and also reported that an experimental group's elevated systolic pressure levels were sustained throughout a 10-week recovery period following termination of conflict. Clearly, caution is necessary when extrapolating from such animal research to humans (see Obrist, 1981; Page, 1977). Nevertheless, results from Lawler's research program, indicating that it is possible to breed animals that develop hypertension when exposed to repeated stress, are consistent with the hypothesis that a genetic susceptibility of this sort may be one route by which hypertension evolves in humans.

Turning to twin studies of blood pressure, Feinleib *et al.* (1975) reported results from 248 monozygotic pairs and 264 dizygotic pairs of adult male twins, aged between 42 and 55 years at the time of examination. The correlation of systolic and diastolic blood pressure levels for the monozygotic twins were 0.55 and 0.58, respectively; for the dizygotic twins the respective values were 0.25 and 0.27. Also, the monozygotic co-twin of a hypertensive was much more likely to be hypertensive than the dizygotic co-twin of a hypertensive (Feinleib *et al.*, 1975). Carroll's group also found high concordance for blood pressure for monozygotic twins; correlations of 0.66 and 0.85 for systolic and diastolic pressure, respectively, were obtained. For the dizygotic twins, the respective coefficients were 0.29 and 0.38 (Sims *et al.*, 1986).

A particularly interesting twin study, in the light of our concerns about the proper interpretation of the Framingham data, is that reported by Schieken and colleagues (Schieken *et al.*, 1989). They found that even at 11 years of age the pattern of monozygotic and dizygotic twin correlations indicate heritabilities (estimates of the proportion of the total phenotypic variance caused by genetic differences between individuals) for systolic and diastolic pressures in the 50% to 60% range, while *no shared environmental effects* were detected. Although correlations are not the best tests of the presence or otherwise of genetic influences (as we shall see later in this chapter), the uniform pattern of higher correlations for monozygotic twins certainly suggests the presence of genetic variance for blood pressure.

Relationship between Offspring Reactivity and Parental Hypertension

Clearly, there appears to be strong evidence of familial aggregation of blood pressure. A second relevant line of inquiry here concerns studies that have examined the relationship between offspring cardiovascular reactivity and parental blood pressure status. The results from these studies provide further inferential evidence of the possible link between reactivity and hypertension development. Epidemiological evidence indicates that the children of hypertensive parents are substantially more likely to develop hypertension themselves than are the children of normotensives (e.g., Paul, 1977). The next question is, do the offspring of hypertensives differ in their cardiovascular reactivity from the offspring of normotensives? This section will provide some evidence that leads us to answer this question with a "yes," although it should be noted that studies failing to find a relationship between offspring reactivity and parental hypertension have certainly been reported (see Muldoon *et al.*, 1993). We shall see that, at least in some studies, the offspring of hypertensives have been found to display the greater reactivity.

Taken together, the implication of these two findings is that heightened cardiovascular reactivity during psychological stressors may be of considerable "etiologic interest" (Manuck & Proietti, 1982). Manuck and Proietti (1982, p. 489) further commented that "it might be hypothesized that for younger individuals carrying a familial predisposition to hypertension, persons who also exhibit a heart rate hyperreactivity to behavioral stressors may be among those who are most likely to develop an essential hypertension in later life." Of course, as already noted, this is presently an inferential argument. Longitudinal studies are needed to provide more definitive answers (longitudinal studies will be discussed in Chapter 10). However, these considerations indicate why considerable research attention has been focused on family history studies. A review of some of them now follows.

Light (1981) reported a study in which attempts were made to obtain family health history information from the parents and the family doctors of subjects who had participated previously in the shock-avoidance reaction time task. Information concerning both parents' blood pressures was obtained for 37 sets of parents. Analysis revealed that both heart rate reactivity and casual systolic blood pressure values were associated with an increased incidence of parental hypertension. Heart rate reactivity, however, showed a much stronger relationship. The highest incidence of parental hypertension was evident in the parents of subjects who displayed mildly elevated casual systolic blood pressure levels and notable heart rate reactivity during the stressor.

Jorgensen and Houston (1981) examined the relationship between parental history of hypertension and cardiovascular response to a shock-avoidance task, mental arithmetic, and the Stroop color-word test. Subjects completed an inventory that elicited health information about both the students themselves and their relatives, and they were classified as having a family history of hypertension if one or both parents had hypertension. As compared with subjects without a history of parental hypertension, subjects with such a history showed reliably greater diastolic blood pressure and pulse rate levels across the stress periods. Jorgensen and Houston (1981) regarded their results as being in line with the hypothesis that consistently excessive sympathetic activity may play a role in the development of sustained hypertension.

Manuck, Giordani, McQuaid, and Garrity (1981) measured subjects' heart rate and systolic blood pressure levels during a prestress baseline period and during a difficult concept-formation task. Subjects were also required to complete a standard family health inventory. Usable inventory data were obtained from 69 subjects, 20 of whom reported a parental history of hypertension. Relative to sons of normotensives, subjects with a hypertensive parent showed significantly higher mean systolic blood pressure levels during the task but not during the pretask baseline period. As regards heart rate, mean heart rate levels during the task did not differ between the two groups of subjects. However, the proportion of hypertensive parents among subjects designated as high heart rate reactors (individuals whose mean heart rate responses to the stressor fell in the upper quartile of such responses) was significantly greater than the corresponding proportion of parents of low heart rate reactors (all remaining subjects).

Manuck and Proietti (1982) explored this issue further using 36 subjects, 18 with and 18 without a parental history of hypertension. Participants were subjected to the same concept-formation task and also a pressurized mental arithmetic task. Offspring of hypertensives exhibited higher mean systolic blood pressure levels than did the sons of normotensives during both tasks, but not during baseline periods. Diastolic blood pressure did not vary reliably with parental status. As regards mean heart rate, the sons of hypertensives showed significantly higher levels than did the sons of normotensives, but this difference occurred in baseline as well as task periods. Subjects in this study also completed an isometric exercise task in which they were required to sustain a handgrip of 30% maximum voluntary contraction on a standard hand dynamometer for 3 minutes. Similar analysis revealed that both mean systolic blood pressure and diastolic blood pressure levels were significantly higher among sons of hypertensive parents. The results for mean heart rates followed the same trend, but the effect was not statistically significant.

As final examples here, two more recent studies by Musante, Treiber, and colleagues are noteworthy. Because the subjects were children, and their parents, therefore, tended to be younger than the parents of college-age subjects employed in other family history studies, family history was defined differently. Both parental and grandparental information was employed in the creation of positive and negative family history of hypertension. Both studies reported significant findings. Musante, Treiber, Strong, and Levy (1990) found that diastolic blood pressure and systemic vascular resistance increases to forehead cold stimulation were significantly greater in subjects with positive family histories of hypertension. Treiber and colleagues (1993) found that positive family history children exhibited greater increases in systemic vascular resistance, systolic blood pressure, and diastolic blood pressure to the forehead cold stressor. (See Murphy, 1992, for a review of the child and adolescent literature with regard to the influence of family history of hypertension.)

These studies provide examples from this line of research. The reader is also directed to recent reviews of this literature (Fredrikson & Matthews, 1990; Lovallo & Wilson, 1992b; Matthews & Rakaczky, 1986). Matthews and Rakaczky (1986) noted from their review that "the studies on physiological reactivity to stress and family history of cardiovascular disease do suggest that important familial factors contribute to individual differences in physiological reactivity" (p. 237).

Some of the available evidence, then, supports the hypothesis that individuals who have a family history of cardiovascular disease exhibit higher reactivity, although there are studies that do not find this relationship (see Muldoon *et al.*, 1993). It should be noted here that the supportive studies have largely used Caucasian American subjects; Anderson *et al.* (1992) recently noted that parallel results have not always been obtained in studies employing African American subjects.

Two comments are appropriate here. First, a weakness of many of the family history studies is that very few verified the parental information, the reports of offspring being taken as sufficient indication of diseases (Matthews & Rakaczky, 1986). Interestingly, while this comment is certainly valid, it is noteworthy that as part of the twin study reported by Carroll *et al.* (1985), they also did a family history study. The full details of this are discussed a little later in this chapter, but the relevant point here is that the parents were actually visited by one of the study's authors (Dr. Jane Sims), who took several blood pressure readings from each parent during her visit. In this way, the authors were able to have high confidence in their categorization of parents as either hypertensive or normotensive. The sons of the hypertensive parents displayed significantly and considerably more cardiac reactivity during a laboratory behavioral challenge than did the sons of the normotensives.

The second comment concerning familial studies is that, once again, while such familial influences on reactivity may be *consistent with* genetic influence, they *do not prove* genetic influence (Rose & Chesney, 1986). Evidence obtained from twin studies is much more compelling, and it is these that we shall now examine.

Cardiovascular Reactivity as a Heritable Predisposing Factor for Hypertension

Several lines of inquiry have led us to suggest the hypothesis that excessive cardiovascular reactivity is part of a heritable predisposition to hypertension. First, there is evidence of metabolically exaggerated cardiac activity during psychological stress, and it has been proposed that these reactions may play a role in the development of hypertension. Second, there is evidence of the stability of individual differences in this regard. Third, there is evidence of familial aggregation for hypertension. Finally, the offspring of hypertensives are more likely to develop hypertension themselves than the offspring of normotensives, and they may also display greater reactivity during psychological stress.

This hypothesis requires a substantial genetic component for variation in cardiovascular reactivity during stress. While other methodologies can hint at evidence for such genetic variation, the twin methodology is able directly to assess the genetic contribution to variation. Before describing one twin study in detail and reviewing several others, a brief overview of the twin study methodology itself is in order.

The Twin Study Methodology

The twin method, which has proved to be one of the most useful techniques for investigating genetic influences on the behavior of humans, makes use of the natural occurrence of identical, or monozygotic, and nonidentical, or fraternal, twins. Monozygotic twins develop from a single fertilized egg, and therefore share the same heredity and have identical genes. Dizygotic twins, on the other hand, develop from different egg cells. Like ordinary siblings, they share, on average, only half of their genes. Studies comparing monozygotic with dizygotic twins help to partition the influence of environment and heredity. If monozygotic twins are more alike in a particular situation than dizygotic twins, part of the variation seen may be due to heritable differences (Jinks & Fulker, 1970). It may also be noted here that, while dizygotic twins share, on average, the same percentage of genes as do ordinary siblings, they are more appropriate for comparison with monozygotic twins than are ordinary siblings because they also share a common interuterine environment, and because they have the same age and parity (Nance, 1984).

Twin Studies of Cardiac Reactivity

As an example of this kind of study, consider the experiment reported by Carroll et al. (1985). While this was not the first twin study to examine cardiovascular reactions to psychological stress, earlier studies had either employed too few subjects, insufficiently sophisticated analytical techniques to afford clear conclusions, or measures not analogous to the reactivity measures used in other recent studies of cardiovascular response to stress (see Turner & Hewitt, 1992, for a review of twin studies). Accordingly, this study employed a large, balanced sample of monozygotic and dizygotic twins along with the powerful test of alternative genetic and environmental models of variation afforded by the statistical technique of weighted least-squares model fitting (see Eaves et al., 1978). The precise details of this analytical technique are not crucial here; the message concerning the evaluation of genetic influence can be stated simply. Also, in the years since this study was completed, behavior genetic analysis has continued to develop and different analytical strategies have become the technique of choice in this research area (see Turner & Hewitt, 1992).

Forty pairs of monozygotic and 40 pairs of dizygotic male twins aged between 16 and 24 years were recruited from the Birmingham Family Study Register. This register was established by the University of Birmingham's (U.K.) Department of Genetics, and it then comprised some 4,500 twin pairs. As far as could be determined from preliminary questioning, none of the 160 twins suffered from any cardiovascular or respiratory disorders. Twin pairs visited the laboratory together. In a letter confirming their appointment, they had been asked to refrain from smoking or drinking tea or coffee for the hour prior to their arrival. On arrival, the reasons for the study and the full experimental instructions were given to both twins together. Order of testing was then decided by the flip of a coin. While one twin completed the experimental task, the other left to complete a battery of questionnaires in a different room. From this point until the end of the experiment, no communication was allowed between the twins.

In the laboratory, subjects were seated in a comfortable armchair in a quiet, modestly lit, temperature-controlled environment. The experimental task was the Space Invaders video game described in Chapter 3. First, a brief practice with the video game was offered to allow subjects to become familiar with the operation of the task. Following this, ECG electrodes were attached, and subjects were asked a final time if they had any questions concerning the task requirements or the experimental protocol; if so, these questions were answered. Subjects then completed the task, following a period of relaxation that was designated the baseline period.

Actually, subjects completed two 8-minute bouts of the video game, each being preceded by a 4-minute relaxation (baseline) period. A heart rate reactivity score was calculated for each task period by subtracting the average heart rate level during the respective preceding baseline period from the average heart rate level during the task period. A comparison of heart rate reactivity during each of the two bouts of the video game indicated considerable consistency of response across time. Temporal stability correlations were calculated (separately for each zygosity) and they averaged 0.76 ($p < .001$) across all subjects (see Carroll et al., 1985). A mean heart rate reactivity score for each subject was then computed as the average of his two reactivity scores. Averaging data across the bouts in this manner thus increased the reliability of the estimate of reactivity for each individual subject without sacrificing important independent aspects of variation.

Initial t-tests conducted on baseline, task, and reactivity data revealed no significant differences between zygosities for any of these values. Interest then focused on the heart rate reactivity scores. While cardiac reactivity was not significantly correlated for the dizygotic twins ($r(38) = 0.11$, NS), a highly significant correlation was found for the monozygotic twins ($r(38) = 0.56$, $p < .001$). This pattern of correlations suggested the presence of genetic variation for heart rate reactivity, but, as noted before, correlational analysis in these circumstances is not the most powerful.

The discipline of behavior genetics has furnished elegant analytical techniques for use in twin studies. On this occasion, weighted least-squares model fitting was employed (see Carroll et al., 1985, for details). The model-fitting procedure attempts to predict the four observed mean squares for heart rate reactivity (a between-family and a within-family mean square for each zygosity). The models of most interest to us were a simple genetic model, which predicts that the ratio of between-family to within-family mean squares will depend on zygosity in a particular way predicted from genetic theory, and a simple environmental model, which predicts that these statistics will not depend on zygosity. As would be expected from the pattern of correlations, the simple genetic model, which hypothesizes additive genetic effects along with those of individual environments, fit the data much better than the simple environmental model. Evidence of a genetic component for variation in heart rate reactivity was thus provided.

To evaluate the size of this genetic component, a heritability estimate was calculated. Heritability can be estimated as the proportion of the total phenotypic variance that is due to genetic differences between individuals. On this occasion, a heritability estimate of 0.48 ± 0.11 was obtained. This indicated that approximately 50% of the variance in heart rate reactivity was of genetic origin. Actually, the value was somewhere between about 40% and 60%; the "± 0.11" indicates our confidence limits.

This is a considerable amount of genetic variation. To put this value of 50% into some kind of perspective, it is worth noting two other heritabilities. For height, heritability is about 90%, and for general cognitive ability (IQ) it is about 0.50 ± 0.20; that is, the heritability estimate is 50% but the error surrounding it may be as high as 20%, so it can only be stated with confidence that the heritability of IQ is between 30% and 70% (Plomin, 1990). Explaining 50% of the variance in reactivity, then, is no small matter.

The next stage of this experiment, as mentioned earlier in the chapter, was to examine the relationship between parental blood pressure and the twins' heart rate reactivity. In all, parental blood pressure was obtained for 59 of the 80 families. Unwillingness to participate on the part of one or both parents, and the unavailability of one or both parents owing to death or separation, precluded data collection for 21 of the families. During each parental visit, the parents completed three questionnaires, and two blood pressure readings were taken using a standard sphygmomanometer and stethoscope, one at the beginning and one at the end of the visit. The blood pressure readings were used to divide the families into two groups: a High Blood Pressure group and a Low Blood Pressure group. To fall into the former category, both parents had to be regarded as having high blood pressure. This necessitated displaying systolic pressures of 140 mmHg or greater and/or diastolic pressures of 90 mmHg or greater on both occasions of measurement, or the taking of antihypertensive medication (determined during the questionnaire phase of the home visits).

Sons of the families in the High Blood Pressure group were then designated the High Parental Blood Pressure group, and sons of families in the Low Blood Pressure group were designated the Low Parental Blood Pressure group. A one-factor ANOVA was then computed using the mean values of each twin pair as data. The High Parental Blood Pressure group displayed an average heart rate reactivity score of 11.6 bpm, while the Low Parental Blood Pressure group displayed a mean of 6.2 bpm $[(F(1,57) = 9.90, p < 0.01)]$. The High Parental Blood Pressure group thus displayed significantly, and considerably, greater average cardiac reactivity.

As a check of the possible influence of parental age here, a similar ANOVA was conducted. The mean age of the two parental groups differed by only 2 years, and the difference was not statistically significant $[(F(1,57) < 1)]$.

This twin study addressed two interrelated propositions. The first proposed a substantial genetic component for variation in heart rate reactivity during psychological stress, and the second predicted that such reactivity would be related to parental blood pressure status. Both hypotheses received support. It was concluded from this study that, while longitudinal studies are necessary to provide an unequivocal test of the overall proposition that marked cardiac reactivity during stress represents a heritable predisposition to developing hypertension, these data are certainly in line with such a proposition (Carroll *et al.*, 1985).

A second twin study conducted at the University of Birmingham (Turner *et al.*, 1986a) did not include a parental visit phase, but it did include two experimental tasks. The video game was again used, but in addition a mental arithmetic task, the MATH task described in Chapter 3 (Turner *et al.*, 1986b), was employed. Because the subject sample was a community sample, and individuals were heterogeneous with regard to numerical skills, this mental arithmetic task proved extremely suitable. Heritability estimates were again calculated for heart rate reactivity scores. On this occasion, a value of 0.61 ± 0.12 was obtained for the video game, and a value of 0.55 ± 0.13 for mental arithmetic (Turner *et al.*, 1986a). These values were of a similar order to that reported for the video game in the previously described twin study.

Twin Studies of Blood Pressure Reactivity

Both of these studies measured only heart rate during psychological challenge. What about twin studies of blood pressure reactivity? There have now been several of these (see Turner & Hewitt, 1992, for detailed comments). For both systolic and diastolic blood pressure, the results are essentially similar to those for heart rate. The literature therefore suggests that cardiovascular reactivity to psychological stress is indeed moderately heritable; the manner in which the cardiovascular system responds to psychological stressors has a sizable genetic component. It appears that the individual's cardiovascular system may be primed for a predetermined level of response in the face of psychological stress (Turner, 1989).

Future Directions of Twin Studies

The future potential for twin studies in cardiovascular behavioral medicine is enormous. Despite the considerable number of reactivity studies employing nontwin subjects that have now been reported, there is a scarcity of twin studies. Turner and Hewitt (1992) reviewed 10 published studies representing the formal reports of 25 years of work in this research domain. Twin studies are more complex to implement since, by definition, they necessitate the recruitment of twins. However, the potential information to be gained will almost certainly make the effort of twin recruitment well worthwhile; twins provide not only all the information that nontwins provide, but also a lot more.

Twin recruitment is certainly easier in institutions that have access to a twin registry, but it can be done in other ways. Ditto (1993) recruited 100 twin pairs in Montreal using a variety of means including advertisement in the media and solicitation through the Montreal Parents of Twins Club. This enabled Ditto to conduct a very elegant study, which will be commented upon further shortly. There have been several statements of the usefulness of twin studies in this area (e.g., Boomsma & Gabrielli, 1985; Plomin & Rende, 1991; Rose & Chesney, 1986), and strong encouragement is hereby given to anyone contemplating the employment of a twin sample.

What avenues of investigation are amenable to examination using behavioral genetic strategies? Blood pressure and heart rate have been examined (though, as stated, by only a very few studies). However, recent advances in the measurement techniques of cardiovascular psychophysiology now permit a much wider range of parameters to be assessed during laboratory experimentation. Cardiac output and total peripheral resistance (see Chapter 3), along with indices of cardiac contractility, are provided by the technique of cardiac impedance, and these physiological parameters are certainly amenable to twin study. Other suitable variables of increasing interest include electrolytes, transmitters, hormones, and receptors (see Schneiderman *et al.*, 1989; Turner *et al.*, 1992).

A second consideration is the need for twin study of minority and female samples; twin studies have not to date focused specifically on such potential group differences in cardiovascular reactivity. Given recent observations that African Americans show larger total peripheral resistance responses in these situations than do Caucasian Americans (see Anderson *et al.*, 1992) (see also Chapter 8), investigation of relative differences in the inheritance of hemodynamic responses in these groups may prove informative. As for gender comparisons, these are only now beginning to be reported. The study reported by Ditto (1993), which was mentioned earlier, is a particularly good exemplar here. Ditto included both male and female monozygotic and dizygotic same-sex twin pairs and also opposite-sex dizygotic twin pairs, thus facilitating the testing of a series of hypotheses concerning the sex limitation of genetic and environmental influences (see Heath *et al.*, 1989).

In addition to using twins in laboratory experimentation, their use in ambulatory studies seems long overdue, especially considering the considerable current interest in ambulatory monitoring (see Chapter 9). To date, the author is aware of only two twin studies involving ambulatory blood pressure monitoring. Rose (1984) reported some preliminary findings on this topic. Although that study was not intended to be a full-blown examination of twins' blood pressure during their daily lives, the preliminary analyses conducted on the limited data available led Rose to comment that "ambulatory records from normotensive twins have value in and of themselves" (Rose, 1984, p. 171). This sentiment is strongly endorsed. The second study was recently reported in abstract form by Alpert *et al.* (1992). In a preliminary analysis of their results from 15- to 17-year-old twins, evidence was found of significant genetic influence on 24-hour blood pressure patterns.

Once ambulatory data are obtained from twins both in the laboratory and also outside the laboratory via ambulatory monitoring, laboratory-field generalization of responses can be studied. Turner and Hewitt (1992) suggested an approach that could fruitfully be applied here. This involves twin laboratory and field data in conjunction with one of the newer behavioral genetic analytical techniques, namely *path analysis* (see Hewitt *et al.*, 1991; Heath *et al.*, 1989). Recently, path analysis has become the technique of choice for research in this area for several reasons, one of which is that it facilitates generalization from univariate to multivariate genetic analysis. While univariate analysis is sufficient to examine laboratory data, if we are interested in relationships between laboratory and ambulatory data, the multivariate analysis is necessary.

Figures 7.1 and 7.2 provide an example of how path analysis can be informative in this context. Imagine a pair of twins, Twin 1 and Twin 2. Figure 7.1 represents the linear path model for a particular pair of phenotypes P1 and P2; these, for example, could represent systolic blood pressure reactivity to a laboratory stressor. Three main influences act upon the phenotypes: These are unobserved genetic influences (A),

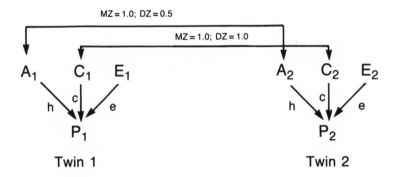

Expectations under the model:

Variance MZ twins : $h^2 + c^2 + e^2$

Covariance MZ twins : $h^2 + c^2$

Variance DZ twins : $h^2 + c^2 + e^2$

Covariance DZ twins : $\frac{1}{2}h^2 + c^2$

Figure 7.1. Univariate path model for the classical twin study. Reprinted, with permission, from Turner & Hewitt, 1992. ©The Society of Behavioral Medicine.

shared environmental (C), and individual environmental (E) influences. The coefficients at the top of Figure 7.1 refer to monozygotic (MZ) and dizygotic (DZ) twin pairs. With regard to genetic influences (A), monozygotic twins receive a coefficient of 1.0 since they are genetically identical, while dizygotic twins receive a coefficient of 0.5 since they share, on average, half their genes. With regard to shared environmental influences (C), both zygosities receive a coefficient of 1.0 since they both have (for argument's sake) identical shared environments if they live together. With regard to individual environmental influences (E), no coefficients are assigned since, as the name suggests, the individual environments are unique to each individual regardless of his or her twin status. Heritability estimates in this case are calculated from the partial regressions h, c, and e according to the following formula:

$$\text{Heritability} = h^2/(h^2 + c^2 + e^2)$$

Figure 7.2 shows how the multivariate approach facilitates the examination of generalization from one setting to another, in this example from laboratory to ambulatory settings. It illustrates a bivariate genetic and environmental model for laboratory (Lab) and ambulatory (Amb) blood pressure. (For simplicity, shared family environments have not been shown here.) In this model we can see genetic effects (Ac, were c = common) that affect both laboratory and ambulatory values. The same is true for common environmental influences (Ec). However, in addition to these, there are new genetic effects that are specific to the ambulatory phenotype (As, where s = specific). The same is true for specific environmental effects (Es). This model can provide a test for the presence of additional genetic and/or environmental influences on ambulatory blood pressure, over and above those on the laboratory phenotypes. The generalization of this path-modeling approach to test multivariate hypotheses is described by Heath *et al.* (1989).

The generalization from laboratory to ambulatory data is just one example of the usefulness and power of path analysis in this context. This area of research is one where associations and interactions between different influences are important. Attention must ultimately be paid to many physiological parameters, cognitive appraisal (the process of situational analysis and assessment that leads to the perception of events as challenging; see Chapter 2), and the interactions between them (Turner, 1989). Hence, the potential for such analysis in cardiovascular behavioral medicine is considerable.

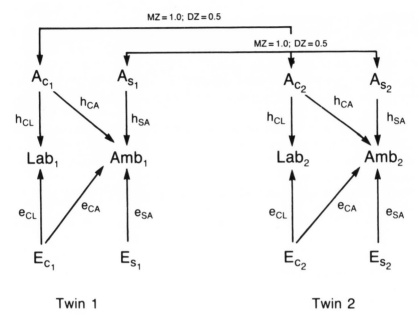

Figure 7.2. An illustrative bivariate path model for the classical twin-study analysis of laboratory and ambulatory measures. Reprinted with permission from Turner & Hewitt, 1992. ©The Society of Behavioral Medicine.

Selective Exposure

One last aspect of behavioral genetic investigation is relevant here. This concerns a concept called *selective exposure*, discussed in several places by Dr. Richard Rose, a long-standing advocate of the use of behavioral genetic techniques in behavioral medicine. Selective exposure is "the transactional process by which people create differences in the environments to which they are exposed and in which they selectively lead their lives" (Rose, 1988, pp. 265–266).

In real life, situations do not just "happen"; individuals actively seek out "opportunities to develop and display the dispositional characteristics that define their individuality (Rose, 1992, p. 95). Just as genetic differences between people contribute to the degree to which they display cardiovascular reactivity, genetic differences influence the degree to which they select life-styles that differ in stress exposure (Rose, 1992). These observations give rise to some interesting speculation. In this volume we are largely concerned with the individual differences—for example, in blood pressure response—that a standard situation elicits from people. In that situation, some individuals will show large responses while others will show minimal change in physiological activation. The implicit assumption is that the high reactor, as compared to the medium or the low reactor, is the one at greatest risk of later cardiovascular disease, since he or she shows the greatest propensity to react. However, this scenario does not pay attention to how likely it is that a particular individual will be exposed to real-life (naturalistic) stressful situations.

Suppose that frequency of exposure to stress is an individual difference dimension under the control of the individual; some people actively seek stressful situations, while others do not. Imagine now that these two individual difference dimensions (cardiovascular reactivity displayed during stress, and propensity to seek out stress) are independent, and that Bill is a high reactor who actively avoids stressful situations whenever possible, whereas Ben is a medium reactor who actively seeks out every challenging situation he can find. From this scenario, it follows that Bill's considerable reactivity will be evoked occasionally, while Ben's medium reactivity will be evoked frequently. The intriguing question here is: Who is at the greater risk, Bill or Ben? A one-time laboratory test (resulting in a greater reactivity score for Bill) would indicate Bill, but somehow something suggests that this might not be the correct answer. Of course, it may be the case that biological predisposition to react to a given extent and the degree to which an individual actively seeks challenge are *not* independent. Either way, the implications are tantalizing.

Summary

This chapter reviewed twin studies examining the genetic origins of individual differences in cardiovascular reactivity and documented evidence that such reactivity is indeed moderately heritable. However, the possibilities for further twin research in this field are enormous. Some suggestions for future study have been made, and examples of useful analytical techniques have been provided. In the opening chapter, the use of psychophysiological strategies in behavioral medicine research was discussed. Accordingly, this chapter has endorsed an approach to the investigation of genetic influence in cardiovascular phenotypes of interest that combines the most recent advances in the measurement techniques of cardiovascular psychophysiology, the experimental paradigms of behavioral medicine, and the analytical techniques of behavioral genetics (Turner & Hewitt, 1992).

Further Reading

1. Carmelli, D., Ward, M.M., Reed, T., Grim, C.E., Harshfield, G.A., & Fabsitz, R.R. (1991). Genetic effects on cardiovascular responses to cold and mental activity in late adulthood. *American Journal of Hypertension, 4,* 239–244.
2. Carroll, D., Hewitt, J.K., Last, K.A., Turner, J.R., & Sims, J. (1985). A twin study of cardiac reactivity and its relationship to parental blood pressure. *Physiology and Behavior, 34,* 103–106.
3. Ditto, B. (1993). Familial influences on heart rate, blood pressure, and self-report anxiety responses to stress: Results from 100 twin pairs. *Psychophysiology,* in press.
4. Ewart, C.K. (1991). Familial transmission of essential hypertension: Genes, environments, and chronic anger. *Annals of Behavioral Medicine, 13,* 40–47.
5. Neale, M.C., & Cardon, L.R. (1992). *Methodology for genetic studies of twins and families.* Dordrecht, The Netherlands: Kluwer Academic Publishers.
6. Plomin, R. (1990). The role of inheritance in behavior. *Science, 248,* 183–188.
7. Plomin, R., DeFries, J.D., & McClearn, G.E. (1990). *Behavioral genetics* (2nd ed.). New York: Freeman.
8. Rose, R.J. (1992). Genes, stress, and cardiovascular reactivity. In J.R. Turner, A. Sherwood, & K.C. Light (Eds.), *Individual differences in cardiovascular response to stress* (pp. 87–102). New York: Plenum.
9. Turner, J.R., Carroll, D., Sims, J., Hewitt, J.K., & Kelly, K.A. (1986). Temporal and intertask consistency of heart rate reactivity during active psychological challenge: A twin study. *Physiology and Behavior, 38,* 641–644.
10. Turner, J.R., & Hewitt, J.K. (1992). Twin studies of cardiovascular response to psychological challenge: A review and suggested future directions. *Annals of Behavioral Medicine, 14,* 12–20.

CHAPTER **8**

Constitutional, Renal, and Personality Factors as Contributors to Individual Differences in Reactivity

In this chapter we shall take a somewhat different approach in examining the phenomenon of individual differences in cardiovascular response to stress. Up to now we have focused very much on the individual subject. Here we shall view that individual as a potential member of various groups. A number of specific constitutional factors have been shown to contribute to individual differences in reactivity in important ways (see Light, 1989); included in this list are age, ethnic or racial group, gender, and aerobic fitness. Unlike the first three factors, we can change our aerobic fitness level, and the relevance of doing so is therefore discussed (it is true that age also changes, but in a manner that is neither under voluntary control nor to the liking of most of us). Also in this chapter we shall look at renal and personality influences on reactivity.

In addition to treating subjects as members of various groups, this chapter also differs from the first three chapters in Part II in that it provides an overview of several research topics, rather than an in-depth analysis of one particular issue. Thus, the same emphasis is not given to discussing precise experimental details. The references contained within the chapter and the readings listed at the end of the chapter (on this occasion broken down into appropriate sections) provide the details of each particular study. However, the studies included here all employed methodologies very similar to those discussed in the previous chapters, and as such it is appropriate to place the present chapter at the end of this section.

Age

Resting (baseline) blood pressure levels show an increase with age, at least in industrial nations (e.g., see Epstein & Eckoff, 1967). This is a widely acknowledged trend that is certainly true in general, even though there will always be individuals whose blood pressure remains relatively constant with increasing years. We mentioned earlier that an often-cited "average" blood pressure was 120 mmHg/80 mmHg. This value is more typical of young, healthy people. It is sometimes said that a systolic value of "100 + age" is a reasonable expectation as people become older, but it should be emphasized that the lower an individual's blood pressure the better.

In keeping with the fact that the majority of our interest in this volume lies with changes from baseline (i.e., reactivity), what is the evidence here? The literature is mixed. Some studies have reported that older adults have shown greater blood pressure increases to standardized stressors, while others have failed to confirm this relationship between age and enhanced blood pressure reactivity (see Light, 1989). On the other hand, the evidence concerning heart rate reactivity appears more consistent. Older adults show less heart rate reactivity than do younger adults.

In addition to comparing the responses of older and young adults, another facet of exploring the influence of age concerns the examination of the responses of children and adolescents (for reviews, see Alpert & Wilson, 1992; Jemerin & Boyce, 1990). Some of the types of studies done using adult samples have also been done using children as subjects. For example, the relationship between cardiovascular reactivity and family history of hypertension has also been explored here. Overall, the results are not dissimilar to those from studies employing adult samples.

Another aspect of studies of reactivity in childhood concerns the relationship between boys' and girls' reactivity. This topic also falls under the umbrella of interest of gender comparisons. For example, evidence is accumulating that boys show greater blood pressure reactivity than do girls (e.g., McCann & Matthews, 1988; Murphy *et al.*, 1986), a finding very much in line with the overall picture for adult gender comparisons (discussed later). However, Matthews and Stoney (1988) examined the influence of age in a group of boys and girls on either side of puberty. The reactions of children in grades 2 through 8 were compared with those in grades 9 through 12. The postpubertal youngsters (grades 9 through 12) showed the same gender differences seen in adult populations, but the prepubertal children did not show any gender differences. This study provided evidence that "reproductive hormones serve, either directly or indirectly, to modulate the magnitude of cardiovascular stress responses" (Stoney, 1992, p. 151). Other researchers have also failed to find gender differences in reactivity in prepubertal children aged 4 to 10 years (Thomas et al., 1984; Treiber et al., 1989).

Ethnic or Racial Comparisons

At present, the major ethnic groups in America are African Americans, Asian Americans, Native Americans, and Hispanic Americans. The 1983 Bureau of the Census report indicated that these groups represented 11.5%, 1.5%, 0.6%, and 6.4% of the population, respectively, in 1980. However, the nation's demographics are changing relatively rapidly, such that the Caucasian American group may well be a minority ethnic group in the future. This is already true at the local level in certain locations in the country.

While cardiovascular disease has a high prevalence in Caucasian Americans, many ethnic groups suffer disproportionately even higher rates (Anderson, 1989). For example, African Americans suffer approximately twice the rate of hypertension. Since this volume focuses on hypertension, and in particular on the possible role of cardiovascular reactivity in the development of hypertension, it is appropriate to examine ethnic differences in reactivity. We shall focus on African–Caucasian comparisons, which is where the majority of work to date has been done. It is hoped that future work will employ other ethnic groups.

Although results from different studies have sometimes been somewhat inconsistent, two observations appear to be relatively robust. Compared with Caucasian Americans, African Americans tend to show the same or *lesser* cardiac reactivity (as indexed by heart rate and cardiac output), and tend to show *greater* vascular reactivity (as indexed by total peripheral resistance). These observations are all the more interesting since different studies have produced differing results concerning which group shows the greater blood pressure responses. For example, Light et al. (1987) found African Americans to exhibit the greater blood pressure responses, while Fredrikson (1986) reported just the opposite. This provides another example of the power of strategies examining the hemodynamic mechanisms operating in a given case.

Evidence of this greater vascular reactivity among African Americans has recently been reported by several authors (e.g., N. B. Anderson et al., 1988; Light & Sherwood, 1989; Light et al., 1993a; Treiber et al., 1990). Their heightened vascular reactivity is particularly evident during the cold pressor task, which (as we noted in Chapter 3) produces a marked vascular vasoconstrictive pattern of reactivity, leading to large increases in total peripheral resistance. This enhanced vascular reactivity in African Americans is of considerable potential interest since hypertension is ultimately a disease of the vasculature, and because they suffer twice the incidence of hypertension compared with Caucasian Americans. The intriguing possibility of a link here awaits further investigation. Confirmation of a possible connection necessitates studies linking total peripheral resistance to disease endpoints (Saab et al., 1992).

What also awaits further investigation is whether different pharmacological interventions in the treatment of hypertension in African and Caucasian Americans might be appropriate. It has been suggested that exaggerated beta-adrenergic drive, leading to blood pressure increases mediated by enhanced heart rate and cardiac output, may be involved in the production of eventual sustained high blood pressure. It seems possible, however, that such sympathetic drive may not be so important in the development of hypertension in African Americans. Exaggerated alpha-adrenergic stimulation, leading to blood pressure increases mediated by enhanced total peripheral resistance, may be of greater relevance. Such speculation has some support from the relatively few studies yet reported that have employed pharmacological blockade studies (see Flamenbaum et al., 1985; Light & Sherwood, 1989). Future research here may prove to be of clinical relevance.

Such information would also be useful at both the individual and group level. While, on the whole, African Americans show greater vascular drive during psychological stress, some Caucasian Americans consistently mediate their blood pressure increases primarily in this manner. Pharmacological intervention that differentiated between dominant hemodynamic mechanisms should therefore be administered ultimately at the individual level.

Finally, much of the research on African–Caucasian American comparisons has employed male subjects. This subject bias was a truism throughout all areas of cardiovascular psychophysiological research until relatively recently (for reasons discussed in the next section, "Gender Comparisons"). This limitation makes statements about female populations somewhat difficult. However, a recent large-scale study (Light *et al.*, 1993a) employed subjects of both races and both genders to facilitate race-gender comparisons. The results for males were in line with the picture already described. Across five different tasks, African American men showed evidence of consistently greater vasoconstrictive responses (higher total peripheral resistance), whereas Caucasian American men demonstrated consistently greater myocardiac (heart rate and cardiac output) reactivity. These differences occurred in the absence of overall blood pressure response differences.

For female subjects, the results indicated more limited and subtle differences. While any differences observed tended to be in the same direction as those evident for male subjects, such differences were only present during certain stressors (Light *et al.*, 1993a). This study therefore highlights the dangers of assuming (either explicitly or, even more insidiously, implicitly) that effects seen in one gender will be occurring commensurately in the other.

For further discussion of this complex issue, the reader is directed to two recent reviews by Anderson and colleagues (Anderson, 1989; Anderson *et al.*, 1992). These are listed at the end of this chapter in the "Further Reading" section.

Gender Comparisons

Epidemiological evidence reveals a gender differential in the prevalence of hypertension. Although males are at greater risk for the development of hypertension during early adulthood, after age 55 the relative risk is reversed, with women showing the greater incidence of disease (Stoney, 1992). Differences in the incidence of disease between any two groups lead to speculation about the potential occurrence of different disease-relevant mechanisms within the groups; the previous discussion of racial differences provided one example of this. The

gender differences in prevalence of hypertension similarly encourage
the investigation of cardiovascular reactivity within both genders.
Again, a brief overview of this area is provided here, and the reader is
directed toward two recent reviews for comprehensive discussions (see
Saab, 1989; Stoney, 1992).

Menstrual Cycle Effects

In a preliminary study employing 24 young adult females and 12
males, Hastrup, Light, and Obrist (1980) found reduced heart rate and
systolic blood pressure responsivity during a reaction time task in the
women tested during the follicular phase of the menstrual cycle as
compared with the women tested during the luteal phase and with the
men. Accordingly, the authors suggested that menstrual cycle phase
may interact with sympathetically mediated cardiovascular responses
to stress. This potential complication led many researchers (the present
author included) to employ male subjects in most of their studies until
menstrual cycle effects became more fully documented. This decision
by some scientists to postpone studies in women led to a lag in our
insights about women's stress responses as compared with those of
men. However, it is fair to note that cardiovascular psychophysiology is
not the only discipline to have focused primary attention on male
subjects in the past. In their book, *The Female Heart: The Truth About
Women and Coronary Artery Disease*, Legato and Colman (1991) describe
how this was true in the medical profession until very recently. For-
tunately, this state of affairs is now changing.

Following the report by Hastrup *et al.* (1980), several other studies
examined potential menstrual cycle effects. Using a similar experimental design, Polefrone and Manuck (1988) found opposite effects, with
women in the follicular phase of the menstrual cycle displaying enhanced blood pressure reactivity compared to women in the luteal
phase.

In a study employing a within-subjects design (the previous two
studies discussed employed a between-subjects design), Carroll *et al.*
(1984) examined the heart rate reactivity of women to a video game task
during both of these phases of their menstrual cycle. Order of testing
(i.e., follicular or luteal phase first) was counterbalanced across subjects. Menstrual cycle phase did not significantly affect cardiac reactivity. Mean heart rate reactivity scores across the 24 subjects (who were
all healthy, reported regular menstrual cycle lengths, and were not

taking contraceptive medication) were 9.6 bpm for the follicular phase and 8.8 bpm for the luteal phase.

A correlation coefficient was then calculated for heart rate reactivity scores on the first and second occasions of testing, irrespective of menstrual cycle phase. A highly significant coefficient of 0.91 was obtained. When the correlation was then computed between follicular and luteal phases rather than occasion of testing, a similar, highly significant coefficient of 0.88 was obtained. Coupled with the very similar mean reactivity scores for the two phases, these results indicated striking stability of individual variations in cardiac reactivity over both time and menstrual cycle phase, leading the authors to suggest the inclusion of females in future studies in this research area (Carroll *et al.*, 1984).

Stoney (1992) observed that at least 12 published studies have investigated the cardiovascular and neuroendocrine responses to stress of women throughout the normal menstrual cycle. The results are disparate and can be somewhat confusing at first. However, as Stoney indicated, grouping these studies by their design (between-subjects or within-subjects) can provide some structure to the results. Although the results of between-subjects designs (testing one group of women in one phase and a second group in the other phase) have been mixed, within-subjects designs (testing the same women in both phases) have generally found that menstrual cycle phase does not significantly influence stress reactivity.

When summarizing all the research done to date, Stoney (1992) concluded that the few effects of menstrual cycle phase reported are small and inconsistent in direction, and that, at least as far as heart rate and blood pressure are concerned, it is likely that the relatively small fluctuations in reproductive hormones that occur during the discrete phases of the menstrual cycle in normally cycling women are not large enough to exert any significant influence on stress responses. Having said this, however, Stoney (1992) added the important caveat that this statement does not necessarily imply that reproductive hormones cannot modulate stress responses in women with abnormal cycles, or that larger magnitude hormonal changes than those occurring in the menstrual cycle cannot modulate reactivity to stress.

Finally, one recent study found that although blood pressure and heart rate responses to stress did not differ across the menstrual cycle, stroke volume and total peripheral resistance responses differed between the luteal phase and follicular phases (Girdler *et al.*, 1993).

Relative to the follicular phase, the luteal phase was associated with significantly greater increases or lesser decreases in stroke volume to all tasks. Conversely, relative to the follicular phase, the luteal phase was associated with significantly greater decreases or lesser increases in total peripheral resistance to all tasks. Coupled with the lack of a difference in blood pressure responses during the two menstrual cycle phases, these results suggest that blood pressure control mechanisms may be different in the follicular and luteal phases (Girdler *et al.*, 1993).

Male-Female Comparisons

Before looking at reactivity comparisons, it is worth noting some gender differences that occur at rest. In general, women display somewhat higher resting heart rates. Women are less heavy, and this higher heart rate is in line with the observation that heart rate increases as body size decreases. This observation holds true across many species. As for blood pressure, women tend to show lower resting blood pressures than do men.

In 1987, Stoney, Davis, and Matthews published a meta-analysis of the results of studies exploring gender differences to date. This analysis revealed that males had relatively greater systolic blood pressure responses to stress, and that females had marginally higher heart rate responses. Since that time other studies have continued this line of research, and in line with previous work, most studies have shown men to have greater overall systolic pressure responses than women (e.g., Light *et al.*, 1993a; Stoney *et al.*, 1988; Weidner *et al.*, 1989; cf. Girdler *et al.*, 1990).

Interestingly, in addition to reporting this difference for task responses, Light *et al.* (1993a) also examined cardiovascular levels during recovery periods following termination of each stressor. Men showed less systolic and diastolic pressure recovery 5 minutes after the end of the tasks than did women. The *recovery* data for diastolic pressure, which showed a gender difference, were particularly compelling because the diastolic *reactivity* data for the genders were very similar.

The study of cardiovascular recovery following stress is a potentially very informative strategy, and one that has not been employed in this field as much as it might have been. In a 5-year follow-up study of borderline hypertensive patients, Borghi *et al.* (1986) found that 100% of the individuals who subsequently developed sustained hypertension had initially shown diastolic blood pressure levels during a mental arithmetic task that did not return to baseline 5 minutes after termination of the task. In contrast, this was true for only 21% of those who did not go on to develop sustained hypertension.

The potential relevance of recovery rate following psychological stress is clear. A given stressor of a given duration may induce the same reactivity in two individuals, but the individual showing the quicker recovery evidences less overall disruption over time of cardiovascular activity. There are also parallels with the study of responses to physical stressors; recovery from a given level of exertion is one index of physical fitness. The further use of recovery measures to investigate "psychological stress fitness" may prove illuminating.

Premenopausal and Postmenopausal Comparisons

A third topic of relevance in this section concerns the comparison of the responses shown by premenopausal and postmenopausal women (see Matthews, 1992). This area of investigation assumes special significance because it is around about the age of menopause that the gender ratio of prevalence of hypertension starts to become reversed. This observation leads to the question of whether the presence of naturally occurring reproductive hormones in premenopausal women is in some way protective against cardiovascular disease. Unfortunately, given the potential importance of this topic, only a few psychophysiological studies have been performed here to date (e.g., von Eiff *et al.*, 1971; Saab *et al.*, 1989).

Saab and colleagues (1989) compared the reactions of similarly aged premenopausal and postmenopausal women during a series of standardized laboratory stressors. One of these tasks was a speech task of the type discussed in Chapter 3, and this task proved particularly informative in this study. The task was a social-evaluative task, and it focused on the evaluation of factors of particular concern to women in midlife, namely appearance and communication skills (Saab, 1989). Other stressors included a mental arithmetic task and a mirror-image tracing task. The results from the study showed that postmenopausal women displayed greater heart rate reactivity across all the tasks. However, in addition, they also displayed greater systolic blood pressure increases during the speech task. Saab *et al.* (1989) noted the importance of using tasks that are relevant for the particular population under study. Because of the potential interaction of type of task (a representation of type of environmental demand) with response patterns, disease-relevant group differences may only be revealed by an appropriate task.

Comparison of Pregnant and Nonpregnant Women

In overviewing the studies comparing the reactivity of premenopausal and postmenopausal women, Stoney (1992) concluded that each of them provided some evidence that reproductive ovarian hormones affect cardiovascular function at rest and/or during stress. We noted earlier that the relatively small fluctuations in hormones during the normal menstrual cycle exerted no consistent influence, and that it may be necessary for hormone levels to be substantial before they exert an influence on cardiovascular reactivity.

Further evidence for this likelihood was recently found by Matthews and Rodin (1992) in a study designed to evaluate the effect on cardiovascular reactivity of the substantial changes in female reproductive hormones that occur during normal pregnancy. A group of women completed laboratory stressors both prior to pregnancy and during the second trimester of pregnancy; a control group of women also completed two testing sessions. While nonpregnant control women's diastolic pressure response did not change across the testing sessions, pregnant women showed a reduced diastolic pressure response (relative to their pre-pregnancy scores) to all laboratory stressors. These results suggested that the heightened levels of reproductive hormones present during pregnancy can mitigate the effects of psychological stress on the cardiovascular system (Matthews & Rodin, 1992). The presently available evidence therefore suggests that the role of endogenous ovarian hormones in moderating cardiovascular reactivity "may likely be a modest but significant one" (Stoney, 1992, p. 157).

Conclusions

This section has provided a starting point for the reader to consider the topic of gender comparisons and to explore the role of ovarian reproductive hormones (both endogenous and exogenous) in the determination of cardiovascular responses to stress. While the current literature does not paint an entirely consistent picture, two conclusions are noteworthy. First, certain gender differences seen in reactivity studies parallel the gender differential for cardiovascular disease observed in industrialized nations including the United States (Saab, 1989). Second, there is little doubt that some forms of ovarian hormones act to modulate the magnitude and pattern of physiological stress responses in certain populations of women (Stoney, 1992). Further research into this area is clearly mandated.

Aerobic Fitness

A variety of evidence suggests that physical activity in general and aerobic exercise in particular reduce the risk of cardiovascular pathology (e.g., Kannel & Sorlie, 1979; Morris et al., 1980; Leon et al., 1987; Paffenbarger et al., 1977, 1984). However, the precise processes by which this protective advantage operates remain unclear. One hypothesis is that aerobic fitness may reduce the physiological impact of psychological stress. If stress-induced physiological activation is of etiological relevance, disease may thus be reduced. This hypothesis is of particular interest in the context of this book, and accordingly we shall examine the evidence. Again, our review will be brief; the reader is referred to de Geus et al. (1990) and Fillingim and Blumenthal (1992) for more detailed overviews.

Studies in this research area can be grouped into two categories—cross-sectional studies and longitudinal studies. The first category contains studies employing between-subjects designs in which the responses of a group of "fit" subjects are compared with the responses of a group of "unfit" subjects. These studies are easier to conduct than are longitudinal studies, but they have the drawback that, even if a relationship between level of fitness and reactivity is found, causality cannot be demonstrated. A third (unknown) factor may cause both aerobic fitness and lower reactivity in the "fit" group. Longitudinal studies, the second category, are harder to conduct, but they circumvent the problem of being unable to ascribe causality in the event of positive findings.

In longitudinal studies, subjects are randomly assigned to exercise programs designed differentially to manipulate levels of aerobic fitness. It is not possible simply to train one group for a period of time and ignore a second group for the same period, and then retest both groups. If a differential decrease in reactivity were then observed, with the exercising group showing the greater attenuation, it could be argued that any intervention may have led to a similar finding. That is, it could be argued that the attention alone lavished on the exercising group in some way caused the effect. Therefore, in addition to incorporating a group that undergoes aerobic training for a given period, longitudinal studies usually include a group (called a control group) that undergoes some other activity known *not* to influence aerobic conditioning, but which otherwise results in this group being treated very similarly to the aerobic training group.

Cross-Sectional Studies

Results from these studies are mixed. Some studies have reported that "fit" individuals compared with "unfit" individuals show lesser cardiovascular reactivity (e.g., Holmes & Roth, 1985; Hull *et al.*, 1984; Turner *et al.*, 1988a; van Doornen & de Geus, 1989), while others found no significant differences between the groups (e.g., Cox *et al.*, 1979; Hollander & Seraganian, 1984; Jamieson & Lavoie, 1987). Of the studies finding an inverse relationship between aerobic fitness and cardiovascular reactivity (i.e., fit subjects showing lower responses), only van Doornen and de Geus (1989) assessed fitness in the most appropriate way with a maximal exercise test (see Fillingim & Blumenthal, 1992), although Turner *et al.* (1988a) employed the method described by Astrand and Rodahl (1977) to estimate maximal oxygen uptake from submaximal heart rate and oxygen consumption data.

Longitudinal Studies

Fillingim and Blumenthal (1992) recently summarized the results from nine longitudinal studies examining the effects of an aerobic conditioning program on cardiovascular reactivity. Again, the literature paints a less than consistent picture. Two studies demonstrated that aerobic exercise moderates stress responses (Blumenthal *et al.*, 1988; Sherwood *et al.*, 1989), and a third showed that while aerobic training did not reduce cardiovascular *reactivity*, it did reduce *absolute levels* of heart rate and blood pressure (Blumenthal *et al.*, 1990). However, some studies reported equivocal results, while others failed to find any effects of aerobic training on cardiovascular responses (e.g, de Geus *et al.*, 1990; Roskies *et al.*, 1986). Thus, overall, the findings from the longitudinal studies are also inconsistent.

De Geus *et al.* (1990) provided a comprehensive discussion of the methodological and conceptual problems involved in the investigation of the effects of aerobic fitness. What at first sight seems to be a clear-cut question that can be asked and answered easily and definitively turns out to be very complex. Even if more studies employing a cross-sectional design show an inverse relationship between fitness and reactivity, the fact that such a design precludes the assignment of causality means that it is possible that relatively high aerobic fitness and relatively low reactivity may simply be "just two different markers of a healthy constitution" (de Geus *et al.*, 1990, p. 459). As for the longitudinal studies, one possibility is that a longer period of aerobic conditioning is needed to induce changes in observed stress reactivity; studies to date have typically employed a training regime of 12 weeks or less. An alternate possibility is that increasing these periods of time would not lead to any greater change in reactivity, even though greater aerobic fitness may be achieved.

Another topic of interest in this research area concerns the effects of single bouts of exercise on physiological responses to challenge and on mood immediately following the exercise. For example, Roy and Steptoe (1991) randomly assigned subjects to three experimental conditions; these were 20 minutes of exercise on a bicycle ergometer at a high level and at a low level, and a 20-minute no-exercise (control) condition. Cardiovascular reactions to mental arithmetic were significantly blunted in the high exercise condition compared with the control condition (Roy & Steptoe, 1991). The literature concerning mood alteration immediately following exercise, another topic of interest, is presently inconsistent. Some studies have reported elevations of mood (Bahrke & Morgan, 1978; Berger & Owen, 1988), while others have failed to confirm these findings (Steptoe & Cox, 1988; Steptoe & Bolton, 1988). However, moderate aerobic conditioning has been found to generate more positive mood changes than do control programs (Moses *et al.*, 1989; Steptoe *et al.*, 1989), indicating that exercise may have direct effects on mood (Roy & Steptoe, 1991).

Aerobic conditioning may alter psychological outlook; increased fitness has been associated with increased "psychological well-being" (Goldwater & Collis, 1985). If this increased fitness leads to increased feelings of self-confidence, fitter subjects may perceive any given situation, including psychophysiological experimental tasks, as less challenging.

Two factors should be considered here. The first can be called the *physical adaptation factor* and the second the *cognitive appraisal factor*. Consider the first factor. Aerobic training may induce physiological adaptations such that a given amount of stress (i.e., a given amount of perceived stress) now has less physiological consequences for cardio-vascular arousal than it did before. The worst outcome here is that there is no effect, since no studies have reported that aerobic conditioning *increases* reactivity. Now consider the second factor, the cognitive appraisal factor. If a given situation is now perceived as less stressful, there will be less psychophysiological reactivity whether the physical adaptation factor came into play or not. The only difference is that there will either be a relatively smaller decrease (less perceived stress, equally sensitive physiological responses) or a relatively larger decrease (less perceived stress and less sensitive physiological responses). Aerobic conditioning, therefore, seems to be a win-win option. As de Geus *et al.* (1990) pointed out, the psychological effects of regular exercise and the physiological effects of aerobic fitness may be mutually reinforcing.

Renal Factors

In the context of the present volume, we are interested in the effects of the central nervous system on renal physiology, particularly during psychological stress. Renal excretory function can be modified by several neural and hormonal factors, including circulatory catecholamines and the renal sympathetic nerves (Falkner & Light, 1986). Both of these factors come into play during stress. Work in this area has been conducted using nonhuman animal models, and it has also employed human subjects in long, complicated, and rigorous experimental protocols.

Evidence from numerous studies indicates that exposing nonhuman animals to stress may result in slowed excretion of a salt load when the animal under study has an inherited or acquired susceptibility toward salt retention (Light, 1992). In work conducted using dogs as subjects, D. E. Anderson and colleagues (Anderson *et al.*, 1987; Anderson *et al.*, 1983) demonstrated that when the animals were exposed for 2 weeks to a combination of high sodium intake (achieved via infusion of saline) and bouts of a shock-avoidance task, the dogs developed a progressive hypertension and evidenced sodium retention but not water retention. In contrast, when the animals received only one of the two conditions (i.e., either infusion of saline only or shock-avoidance tasks only), there was no increase in blood pressure and no sodium retention occurred. As Light (1992) observed, these studies "provided clear evidence that stress exposure plays an essential and causal role, as did the increased sodium intake, in the development of this hypertension" (p. 250).

As for studies evaluating the effect of behavioral stress on sodium excretion in man, there have been relatively few (for a recent review see Light, 1992). Of interest have been the effects of different diets on reactivity, and the possible role of psychological stress in inducing sodium and fluid retention in certain individuals (see Light *et al.*, 1983). The practical side of running such studies is very complex, and many factors (such as prior dietary intake of sodium and potassium) need to be carefully controlled. One way to do this is to admit experimental subjects as inpatients for a certain length of time before the stress testing occurs. In this way, their diets can be strictly controlled by providing them with meals prepared under the guidance of a nutritionist.

Despite their inherent demands, some very interesting investigations of the effects of differing dietary intakes of sodium have been reported. However, thus far their results have not led to a clear overall picture (Light, 1992). One reason for this may be the relatively short periods of dietary manipulation. Future studies may address this. They may also address the effects of increasing dietary intake of potassium as one means of combatting the effects of higher sodium intakes; the ratio of potassium and sodium intake appears to be important in determining blood pressure (see Meneely & Battarbee, 1976). Attention may also need to focus on other substances—for example, calcium and magnesium—to understand fully the stress-sodium interaction. Because the kidneys are one of the interactive systems involved in blood pressure regulation, cardiovascular behavioral medicine must continue to integrate knowledge of their influence into its overall description of the effects of stress on cardiovascular function.

Personality Characteristics

In this section we shall focus on personality characteristics that may influence reactivity, and which therefore may play a role in the etiology of cardiovascular disease via their influence on reactivity. In this context, personality characteristics can be thought of as those "thoughts, feelings, motives, and behaviors that serve to identify or distinguish a person" (Houston, 1992, p. 104). While short-lived personality characteristics are important in their own right, attention will focus on enduring personality characteristics. Cardiovascular disease develops over an extended time frame, and therefore if such personality factors are to be implicated in the overall etiological process they need to be relatively durable (Houston, 1992).

Houston (1992) presented a cognitive model of how personality characteristics can exert influence on physiological arousal via their influence on emotional arousal and motivational arousal. This model is reprinted here as Figure 8.1. A key feature of this model is the interactive nature of the components, and it illustrates well the important point that personality characteristics do not influence reactivity (i.e., physiological arousal) directly, or relate to cardiovascular disease directly; rather, they do so in the context of other variables and processes (Houston, 1992). This model complements the overall model presented at the end

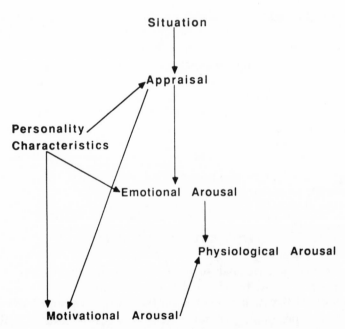

Figure 8.1. A model of emotional, motivational, and physiological arousal. Reprinted with permission from Houston, 1992. ©Plenum Press.

of Chapter 2 (Figure 2.5), extending the ideas summarized in the first unit of that model. We shall briefly examine some of the personality characteristics that have been studied in this context; the reader is referred to Houston (1989, 1992) for more detailed and comprehensive coverage.

Some personality characteristics influence the appraisal process (which, as we have noted already several times in this volume, is the starting point of the entire process of interest here). One characteristic of interest is locus of control (see Rotter, 1966). This characteristic has two levels—internal and external control. Internal control refers to people's beliefs that desired end-results can be achieved as a direct result of their own efforts, while external control refers to beliefs that outcomes are largely the result of chance, fate, or the actions of other, powerful individuals. Generally, greater cardiovascular reactivity has been shown by subjects with an internal locus of control (Houston, 1972; Manuck *et al.*, 1978), possibly because they become more involved in the situation, believing that they can influence its outcome.

Another characteristic that influences appraisal is cynical mistrust. Whether other people are believed to be trustworthy and supportive or untrustworthy and hostile influences an individual's situational appraisals (Lazarus, 1966). Cynical mistrust is often measured by the Cook and Medley (1954) Hostility Scale. Research employing the hostility scale has revealed a very interesting three-way interaction among hostility, reactivity, and the specific situation. Suarez and Williams have examined the relationship between reactivity and hostility. In one study (Suarez & Williams, 1989), subjects were classified as high hostile or low hostile according to their scores on the Cook and Medley Hostility Scale. They were then randomly assigned to one of two conditions— harassment or nonharassment. In the nonharassment condition, subjects simply completed an anagram task. In the harassment condition, the technician running the study harassed subjects during their completion of the task with phrases such as "Stop mumbling; I can't understand your answers!" Compared to the nonharassment condition, the harassment condition led to increased cardiovascular arousal. However, the discrepancy between conditions was greater for the high hostile subjects than for the low hostile subjects.

This study again illustrates the fact that when examining a particular issue (in this case hostility), appropriate task conditions must be employed. The element of harassment made all the difference here as compared with the straightforward anagram task. To underscore this

point, it is worth noting that hostility scale scores have not been found
to be related to reactivity for laboratory tasks that are not associated
with conflict or harassment (e.g., Kamarck *et al.*, 1990; Smith &
Houston, 1987).

Further examination of dimensions of hostility can be found in
several recent papers (e.g., Suarez & Williams, 1990; Suarez *et al.*, 1991;
Smith *et al.*, 1991).

Other personality characteristics that have been examined, to a
greater or lesser degree, are anxiety, anger, reactive or expressive
hostility, power motivation, dominance, and competitiveness (see
Houston, 1992). In addition to considering each of these individually,
multifaceted constructs encompassing several characteristics, such as
the Type A behavior pattern, can be studied. Then, characteristics that
modulate emotional and motivational arousal, such as temperament
and coping style, need to be studied, as does the interaction between
different personality characteristics.

While this area of research is complex, two simple guidelines can
be suggested when studying the relationships between personality
characteristics and cardiovascular reactivity. First, it is very important to
select or create "experimental arrangements" (Houston, 1992) that actually engage the personality characteristics under study. Second, *interactions* among personality, biology, and specific situations need to be paid
particular attention. Certain personality characteristics will only be
engaged by certain situations, and the resulting cognitive arousal may
only impact on certain biologically predisposed individuals to produce
cardiovascular arousal.

Summary

This chapter summarized several lines of investigation concerning
potential group differences in cardiovascular response to stress. The
effects of age, ethnicity, gender, and aerobic fitness were examined.
Each of these factors exerts certain influences upon reactivity.

Renal factors and personality characteristics were also considered.
Both of these topics are complex. In the first case, it appears that longer
dietary interventions may be necessary to evaluate more thoroughly the
effects of dietary sodium on cardiovascular function. Also, attention
should be paid to potassium, calcium, and magnesium to understand
more fully the stress-sodium interaction. As regards personality charac-

teristics, individual characteristics, multifaceted constructs that encompass several characteristics, and interactions between different characteristics all need to be considered. Also, interactions among personality, biology, and specific situations are particularly important.

Further Reading

Age

1. Alpert, B.S., & Wilson, D.K. (1992). Stress reactivity in childhood and adolescence. In J.R. Turner, A. Sherwood, & K.C. Light (Eds.), *Individual differences in cardiovascular response to stress* (pp. 187–201). New York: Plenum.
2. Lawler, K.A., & Allen, M.T. (1981). Risk factors for hypertension in children: Their relationship to psychophysiological responses. *Journal of Psychosomatic Research, 23,* 199–204.
3. McCann, B.S., & Matthews, K.A. (1988). Influences of potential for hostility, Type A behavior, and parental history of hypertension on adolescents' cardiovascular responses during stress. *Psychophysiology, 25,* 503–511.
4. Matthews, K.A., Manuck, S.B., & Saab, P.G. (1986). Cardiovascular responses of adolescents during a naturally occurring stressor and their behavioral and psychophysiological predictors. *Psychophysiology, 23,* 198–209.
5. Treiber, F.A., Musante, L., Strong, W.B., & Levy, M. (1989). Racial differences in young children's blood pressure. *American Journal of Diseases of Children, 143,* 720–723.

Ethnic or Racial Differences

1. Anderson, N.B. (1989). Ethnic differences in resting and stress-induced cardiovascular and humoral activity: An overview. In N. Schneiderman, S.M. Weiss, & P.G. Kaufmann (Eds.), *Handbook of research methods in cardiovascular behavioral medicine* (pp. 433–451). New York: Plenum.
2. Anderson, N.B., McNeilly, M., & Myers, H. (1992). Toward understanding race difference in autonomic reactivity: A proposed contextual model. In J.R. Turner, A. Sherwood, & K.C. Light (Eds.), *Individual differences in cardiovascular response to stress* (pp. 125–143). New York: Plenum.
3. Light, K.C., & Sherwood, A. (1989). Race, borderline hypertension and hemodynamic responses to behavioral stress before and after beta-adrenergic blockade. *Health Psychology, 8,* 577–595.
4. Light, K.C., Turner, J.R., Hinderliter, A., & Sherwood, A. (1993). Race and gender comparisons: I. Hemodynamic responses to a series of stressors. *Health Psychology, 12,* 354–365. [This paper is also of relevance for the next section.]
5. Saab, P.G., Llabre, M.M., Hurwitz, B.E., Frame, C.A., Reineke, L.J., Fins, A.I., McCalla, J., Cieply, L.K., & Schneiderman, N. (1992). Myocardial and peripheral vascular responses to behavioral challenges and their stability in black and white Americans. *Psychophysiology, 29,* 384–397.

Gender Comparisons

1. Girdler, S.S., Turner, J.R., Sherwood, A., & Light, K.C. (1990). Gender differences in blood pressure control during a variety of behavioral stressors. *Psychosomatic Medicine, 52*, 571–591.
2. Matthews, K.A. (1992). Myths and realities of the menopause. *Psychosomatic Medicine, 54*, 1–9.
3. Saab, P.G. (1989). Cardiovascular and neuroendocrine responses to challenge in males and females. In N. Schneiderman, S.M. Weiss, & P.G. Kaufmann (Eds.), *Handbook of research methods in cardiovascular behavioral medicine* (pp. 453–481). New York: Plenum.
4. Stoney, C.M. (1992). The role of reproductive hormones in cardiovascular and neuroendocrine function during behavioral stress. In J.R. Turner, A. Sherwood, & K.C. Light (Eds.), *Individual differences in cardiovascular response to stress* (pp. 147–163). New York: Plenum.
5. van Doornen, L.J.P. (1986). Sex differences in physiological reactions to real life stress and their relationship to psychological variables. *Psychophysiology, 23*, 657–662.

Aerobic Fitness

1. Blumenthal, J.A., Emery, C.F., Walsh, M.A., Cox, D.R., Kuhn, C.M., Williams, R.B., Jr., & Williams, R.S. (1988). Exercise training in healthy Type A middle-aged men: Effects on behavioral and cardiovascular responses. *Psychosomatic Medicine, 50*, 418–433.
2. de Geus, E.J.C., van Doornen, L.J.P., de Visser, D.C., & Orlebeke, J.F. (1990). Existing and training induced differences in aerobic fitness: Their relationship to physiological response patterns during different types of stress. *Psychophysiology, 27*, 457–478.
3. Fillingim, R.B., & Blumenthal, J.A. (1992). Does aerobic fitness reduce stress responses? In J.R. Turner, A. Sherwood, & K.C. Light (Eds.), *Individual differences in cardiovascular response to stress* (pp. 203–217). New York: Plenum.
4. Holmes, D.S., & Roth, D.L. (1985). Association of aerobic fitness with pulse rate and subjective responses to psychological stress. *Psychophysiology, 22*, 525–529.
5. van Doornen, L.J.P., de Geus, E.J.C., & Orlebeke, J.K. (1988). Aerobic fitness and the physiological stress response: A critical evaluation. *Social Science and Medicine, 26*, 303–307.

Renal Factors

1. Anderson, D.E., Kearns, W.D., & Worden, T.J. (1983). Potassium infusion attenuates avoidance-saline hypertension in dogs. *Hypertension, 5*, 415–420.
2. Falkner, B., & Light, K.C. (1986). The interactive effects of stress and dietary sodium on cardiovascular reactivity. In K.A. Matthews, S.M. Weiss, T. Detre, T.M. Dembroski, B. Falkner, S.B. Manuck, & R.B. Williams, Jr. (Eds.), *Handbook of stress, reactivity, and cardiovascular disease*, (pp. 329–341). New York: Wiley.
3. Grignolo, A., Koepke, J.P., & Obrist, P.A. (1982). Renal function, heart rate, and blood pressure during exercise and avoidance in dogs. *American Journal of Physiology, 242*, R482–R490.

4. Light, K.C. (1992). Differential responses to salt-stress interactions: Relevance to hypertension. In J.R. Turner, A. Sherwood, & K.C. Light (Eds.), *Individual differences in cardiovascular response to stress* (pp. 245–263). New York: Plenum.
5. Light, K.C., & Turner, J.R. (1992). Stress-induced changes in the rate of sodium excretion in healthy black and white men. *Journal of Psychosomatic Research, 36,* 497–508.

Personality Characteristics

1. Houston, B.K. (1992). Personality characteristics, reactivity, and cardiovascular disease. In J.R. Turner, A. Sherwood, & K.C. Light (Eds.), *Individual differences in cardiovascular response to stress* (pp. 103–123). New York: Plenum.
2. Lazarus, R.S., & Folkman, S. (1984). *Stress, appraisal, and coping.* Berlin: Springer-Verlag.
3. Smith, T.W., McGonigle, M., Turner, C.W., Ford, M.H., & Slattery, M.L. (1991). Cynical hostility in adult male twins. *Psychosomatic Medicine, 53,* 684–692.
4. Suarez, E.C., & Williams, R.B., Jr. (1989). Situational determinants of cardiovascular and emotional reactivity in high and low hostile men. *Psychosomatic Medicine, 51,* 404–418.
5. Ward, M.M., Chesney, M.A., Swan, G.E., Black, G.W., Parker, S.D., & Rosenman, R.H. (1986). Cardiovascular responses of type A and type B men to a series of stressors. *Journal of Behavioral Medicine, 9,* 43–49.

PART **III**

*Everyday Reactivity and Risk
for Cardiovascular Disease*

CHAPTER 9

Laboratory-Field Generalization
of Cardiovascular Activity

In Chapter 5 we noted the three attributes of individual differences in reactivity that have particular significance when considering current hypotheses that link cardiovascular reactivity to aspects of cardiovascular disease (Manuck *et al.*, 1989). These were temporal stability, intertask consistency, and laboratory-field generalization. The first two of these attributes were dealt with in detail in that chapter. Accordingly, we will now examine laboratory-field generalization.

Laboratory stressors can be thought of as representations of real-life stressors. It is much easier to conduct tightly controlled experiments in a psychophysiological laboratory than in people's natural, everyday environments. However, it is people's cardiovascular activity in normal situations that is ultimately of importance. If cardiovascular reactivity does play a role in the etiology of hypertension and/or coronary heart disease, it will have its effects in the periods when individuals are exposed to stressful situations in daily life. Thus, a crucial question is: Do those people who show large responses to laboratory stressors also show exaggerated responses to naturally occurring stressors met in daily life? Put another way, it is important to determine whether the individual differences in reactivity in the laboratory predict measurements made in the real world. This is what is meant by laboratory-field generalization.

The temporal stability of individual differences in laboratory reactivity has, as seen in Chapter 5, typically been investigated with correlational techniques. Reactivity scores are obtained during two laboratory sessions, and scores on Test 1 are compared in a correlational analysis with scores on Test 2. This same type of experimental strategy has been employed in the investigation of laboratory-field generalization. In this case, reactivity scores obtained during laboratory testing are correlated with reactivity scores obtained from a period of real-world measurement.

This avenue of investigation, however, brings with it a collection of methodological problems that do not occur in laboratory experimentation. Because of the difficulties, a different analytical technique, *regression analysis*, can sometimes reveal relationships that might otherwise be obscured by confounding influences. In the real world, people talk, walk, change posture, and eat meals. All of these activities influence cardiovascular parameters, and thus they can make it difficult to uncover the cardiovascular effects caused specifically by real-life stressors. In this chapter we shall look at experiments that have investigated laboratory-field generalization in various ways, but first it may be useful to describe how real-life cardiovascular measurements are made.

Ambulatory Monitoring

Ambulatory monitoring is the name often given to the process of recording subjects' cardiovascular activity (or other physiological activity) while they are outside the laboratory, conducting their business. Typically, subjects come to the laboratory early in the day, where they are fitted with portable measuring devices. These are lightweight recorders designed to interfere as little as possible with normal activities. With specific exceptions, such as swimming and taking a shower, most daily activities can be done with minimal interference.

Some ambulatory monitors record heart rate information. One example is the Oxford MR-10 Medilog Tape Recorder, which is made of lightweight aluminum, powered by small batteries, and carried in a leather pouch supported by a waist belt. It records electrocardiogram signals on conventional audiocassettes. To obtain heart rate information, the tape recordings can be processed by computer systems that can produce minute-by-minute statements of heart rate (e.g., see Turner & Carroll, 1985b).

Other monitors can record blood pressure in ambulatory settings. Two examples are the Accutracker and the Spacelabs monitors (see Light *et al.*, 1988). These monitors automatically inflate and deflate the arm cuff that is worn by subjects, determine systolic and diastolic pressures, and store these readings in a memory unit until they can be downloaded sometime after the subject returns the monitor. The monitors can be preprogrammed to take readings at regular intervals (for example, every 20 minutes). They can also be programmed to take readings on a quasi-random basis. In this case, they are taken on average every 20 minutes, for example, but the length of time between two consecutive readings varies randomly. The advantage of this strategy is that the subject cannot anticipate exactly when the reading will occur, and therefore cannot deliberately alter his or her activity accordingly. Subjects are usually asked to keep their arm still for the duration of each reading. However, if they happen to be doing something that prevents them from keeping their arm still for a particular reading (e.g., they are driving through very busy traffic), subjects are instructed not to alter their behavior on that occasion of measurement.

Thus far we have looked at the technical side of ambulatory monitoring to discuss the monitors that provide the physiological data. In the experiments of interest in this book, however, there is another equally important aspect to ambulatory monitoring. This concerns the behavioral assessment of subjects' activities during the day, or more specifically at the times at which the readings were taken. We need to know what people were doing at each occasion of measurement so that, at the simplest level, we can determine whether they were "stressed" or "unstressed" at that moment. This behavioral information, however, is also of use in disentangling other real-world influences on cardiovascular activity (i.e., influences that are not psychological stressors). Influences in this category include physical activity, posture, and consumption of caffeine, nicotine, and food. It can also be helpful to know the subject's location (e.g., at home or at work). To help subjects provide a standardized report on their activity at each occasion of measurement, behavioral diaries have been developed (see Chesney & Ironson, 1989; Van Egeren & Madarasmi, 1988). Each time a reading occurs, the subject completes a page in a booklet of identical pages when the cuff has deflated.

Before continuing to look at the use of ambulatory data in studies examining laboratory-field generalization of reactivity, it should be made clear that ambulatory monitoring is an investigative technique in its own right. It is of great interest to the medical community to know how blood pressure behaves during the course of a day. Average blood pressures may be calculated for the hours spent at work, at home, and asleep. Variability in blood pressure readings obtained in each of these categories may also be of considerable interest. There is increasing evidence that, compared with standard clinic and laboratory measurements, ambulatory monitoring provides a more representative assessment of an individual's cardiovascular functioning (Chesney & Ironson, 1989). For example, evidence shows that ambulatory blood pressure levels, especially during work periods, are better predictors of hypertensive complications and mortality than are causal office measurements (Devereux et al., 1983; Perloff et al., 1983). For more information on ambulatory monitoring, it is suggested that readers start with the work of Harshfield, James, Mancia, Parati, and Pickering (see Harshfield & Pulliam, 1992; James et al., 1988; Mancia et al., 1993; Pickering, 1991a).

Laboratory-Field Generalization

Laboratory-field studies can adopt two basic approaches. The laboratory phase is the same in each case, but the real-life assessments are different. One approach is for experimenters to select one particular naturalistic stress and to obtain ambulatory measures when it occurs. The second is the open-ended approach, where subjects simply go about their normal daily activity.

Studies Employing a Specific Naturalistic Stressor

In a study conducted several years earlier and reported in 1988, Obrist and Light examined the heart rate responses of 18 subjects in the laboratory and in two naturally occurring real-life situations, attending a class (the low-stress, real-life period) and taking an examination (the high-stress, real-life period). On the basis of their responses during the laboratory reactivity testing, subjects were divided into high heart rate and low heart rate reactors. The heart rates of these two groups were then examined for both real-world situations. The heart rates of the low reactors were similar during both real-world periods, while the heart rates of the high reactors were appreciably greater during the high-stress period (the exam) than during the low-stress period. The authors concluded that these data suggested that the challenge of an exam influenced heart rate only in the subjects who showed the greater heart rate reactivity in the laboratory (Obrist & Light, 1988).

In a study reported by Turner et al. (1987a), 24 subjects completed two laboratory challenges. Average heart rate reactivity scores across the two tasks were taken and then used to select the three highest and the three lowest reactors. These six subjects then took part in the second phase of the study, which consisted of a public-speaking competition. In this category of laboratory-field studies, the real-world phase is deliberately and specifically chosen to incorporate a situation generally regarded as stressful. Public speaking certainly meets this criterion. Whether giving a speech in front of a large audience, having a job interview before a select panel, or asking a boss in private for a raise, interpersonal communication in an evaluative context is a common and stressful experience for us all (Turner, 1989).

On this occasion, the speaking competition was structured as a "balloon debate." Subjects participated in pairs (each pair consisting of a high reactor and a low reactor). Each pair sat on chairs in front of an audience, consisting of the other 18 subjects from the original pool of 24 who completed the laboratory phase of the study. A balloon debate works by pretending that the two participants are in a hot-air balloon that is damaged and losing height while flying over very dangerous terrain. All available ballast has already been jettisoned, and, if nothing else is done, the balloon will undoubtedly crash and both occupants will die. All that remains possible in order to save at least one life is for one person to jump, thereby guaranteeing the life of the other! The two individuals engage in a speaking competition for 10 minutes, with the audience deciding at the end who should "jump." During the 10-minute debate, subjects' heart rates were monitored using Oxford MR-10 Medi-log recorders. These heart rate task levels were later used in conjunction with real-world baseline levels to compute real-world reactivity scores. Real-world baseline data were collected by asking subjects to wear the monitors at home, and to record 10 minutes of data while relaxing there.

Results from this study are shown in Table 9.1. It can be seen that, with one notable exception (subject 17, to whom we shall return in a moment) the three high heart rate reactors (as defined by the laboratory session) showed substantial real-world reactivity scores, and that the low reactors showed much less response. The exception was a subject who appeared enormously reactive to the balloon debate speaking task, but unreactive to the laboratory stressors. However, closer inspection of the data revealed the source of this apparent discrepancy between laboratory and real-world responses.

Although subject 17's task levels in both situations were very similar (87.9 and 91.3 bpm for laboratory and real world, respectively),

Table 9.1. Heart Rates (bpm) during Each Condition for the
Subjects Chosen for the Public-Speaking Competition

	Laboratory			Real world		
Subject	Baseline	Task	Reactivity	Baseline	Task	Reactivity
Low reactors						
8	70.2	68.3	−1.9	65.2	73.2	8.0
12	72.5	72.4	−0.1	86.3	91.5	5.2
17	89.0	87.9	−1.1	46.8	91.3	44.5
High reactors						
15	83.8	99.8	16.0	75.9	105.3	29.4
16	62.0	80.3	18.3	72.2	86.5	14.3
22	67.3	84.6	17.3	68.3	100.7	32.4

Note: Laboratory data are averaged across video game and mental arithmetic laboratory tasks.
Reprinted with permission from Turner *et al.*, 1987. ©Elsevier Science Publishers B.V. (Biomedical Division).

his baseline values were very different; his laboratory resting baseline was 89.0 bpm, while his real-world baseline value was 46.8 bpm. (This discrepancy was so large that a second real-world baseline was obtained for this subject; a value extremely close to the original 46.8 bpm was obtained.) Thus, it appears that what was really happening was that, far from being a low reactor, this subject was an extremely high reactor, but he was reacting to the entire laboratory experience. Just being in the laboratory caused his heart rate to increase somewhere around 40 bpm, and when the task demands were superimposed on top of this no real extra change was observed.

This point serves as an illustration of the problem of obtaining reliable baseline data. This process requires allowing subjects to relax as much as possible in a laboratory environment, which, by its very nature, can cause a certain amount of stress, and thus stress-induced cardiovascular activation. This problem is analogous to the phenomenon of "white coat hypertension," where patients appear to have higher blood pressure levels when measured in the formal environment of a doctor's office than when measured at home (e.g., see Pickering *et al.*, 1988).

Returning to the balloon debate, the results suggested that the extent of heart rate reactions to real-world behavioral challenge may be indicated by the magnitude of reaction shown to laboratory challenges (Turner *et al.*, 1987a). This conclusion is strongly tempered by a very small sample size (only six subjects took part in both laboratory and field phases), and the resulting absence of formal statistical evaluation of the laboratory-field association. However, this study certainly hints at the presence of such an association, and it serves as an example of the kind of small-scale study that a reader may wish to undertake as part of a course's experimental requirements.

In other examples of studies in this category, the specific naturalistic stressor has been the anticipation of an evaluated musical performance (Abel & Larkin, 1991), the public defense of a doctoral thesis (van Doornen & van Blokland, 1992), and giving a speech in an English class (Matthews *et al.*, 1986a).

Open-Ended Ambulatory Studies

In studies falling into this category, subjects go about their normal daily activity. Ambulatory monitoring sometimes occurs during waking hours only, or it may also occur during sleep. Again, we shall look at two examples.

Turner and Carroll (1985b) tested the heart rate reactivity of 31 subjects to a video game task, and also monitored each subject's heart rate ambulatorily for an 8-hour period. During the ambulatory period, subjects kept a detailed written account of their behavior using a behavioral diary. They were asked to record the time and character of any change in their activity or behavior throughout the 8 hours of monitoring. In addition, they were taught a simple code for categorizing their activity at any time: A = low physical, low mental activity; B = low physical, high mental activity; C = high physical, low mental activity; and D = high physical, high mental activity.

Real-world heart rate reactivity was defined as the difference between average heart rate during samples of low physical, high mental activity (category B) and average heart rate during samples of low physical, low mental activity (category A). In this manner, category B activities were regarded as the "real-world task" period, and category A activities as the "real-world baseline" period. Real-world reactivity scores correlated significantly with reactivity to the laboratory video game task, providing evidence for laboratory-field generalization of heart rate response.

Next, consider the study conducted by Parati *et al.* (1988). They found an interesting and significant relationship between blood pressure reactivity to a mirror-drawing laboratory task and blood pressure variability during daytime ambulatory monitoring. Indeed, the correlation coefficient they obtained (0.72) is particularly noteworthy in this research domain.

Several experiments have employed blood pressure variability as their real-world measure, instead of using real-world reactivity measures. The apparently simple designation of "baseline" and "task" periods (to use laboratory terminology) is not always straightforward. First, consider real-world baseline determination. Because some subjects may not relax completely at all during a day of ambulatory monitoring, various strategies to obtain a "baseline" have been employed. These include having the subject rest in the laboratory just prior to commencement of ambulatory monitoring, using previously obtained laboratory baselines, and using measurements taken while the subject is asleep.

Second, the designation of the real-world "task" period can be even more difficult. In contrast to the laboratory, where the start and the end of stressor tasks are very clear, the precise onset and termination of real-world stressors can be difficult, if not actually impossible, to determine. Accordingly, variability measures in ambulatory data have been used instead of reactivity scores on some occasions. All other things being equal, it is likely that the more reactive individual will show greater variability, since there will be more of a change in cardiovascular activity each time a stressor is met.

An Overview of Correlational Studies

In the above categories, examples that reported positive findings were deliberately chosen. At this point, however, it should be made clear that several other studies have not reported significant laboratory-field associations. Indeed, the picture painted by the current laboratory-field generalization literature can be quite confusing at first sight. Rather than look at a lot of individual studies, therefore, a brief overview is provided here. The reader is encouraged to obtain further details from four recent reviews: Johnston et al. (1992); Turner et al. (1993c); van Doornen and Turner (1992); and Van Egeren and Gellman (1992).

To acquire an overall feel for the studies of laboratory-field generalization that have employed correlational strategies, it is possible to categorize studies according to various criteria (see van Doornen & Turner, 1992). We have already seen one grouping (i.e., studies employing a specific naturalistic stressor and studies employing open-ended ambulatory monitoring). The four categories presented below are created in a manner that is *completely independent* from the specific stressor/ open-ended monitoring classification. Accordingly, studies in both of these categories can also fall into any of the following four categories:

1. Studies using laboratory reactivity scores to predict ambulatory reactivity scores (i.e., studies investigating correlational associations between laboratory and field reactivity).
2. Studies using laboratory reactivity scores to predict ambulatory mean levels (in open-ended studies, "work" and "home" mean levels, and also perhaps "asleep" mean levels, may be considered separately).
3. Studies using laboratory task levels (i.e., absolute levels) to predict ambulatory reactivity scores.
4. Studies using laboratory task levels to predict ambulatory mean levels.

In keeping with the central theme of this volume (i.e., cardiovascular reactivity), it is logical to presume that our interest might focus initially on studies in the first of these four categories. However, while there are certainly exceptions, the literature does not provide consistent evidence for a relationship between laboratory and ambulatory reactivity. There is also a lack of consistent evidence for an association between laboratory reactivity and ambulatory mean levels. The strongest consistently observed relationships in correlational laboratory-field studies are between laboratory and ambulatory mean levels (i.e., studies in the fourth category).

This lack of a consistent association between laboratory reactivity and real-world cardiovascular activity appears at first sight to be quite disconcerting. It seems to indicate that laboratory reactivity is not able to predict cardiovascular activity in nonlaboratory settings. However, several considerations are pertinent here. We have already noted that the designation of real-world "baseline" and "task" levels can be difficult. This in turn means that obtaining reliable real-world reactivity scores can be problematic. Therefore, it may be a better strategy to examine relationships between laboratory reactivity and ambulatory *levels* of cardiovascular activity.

Two considerations support this strategy. First, the assessment of ambulatory levels, unlike ambulatory reactivity, is not problematic. Second, ambulatory levels, as noted earlier, are themselves predictors of hypertensive complications and mortality (Devereux *et al.*, 1983; Perloff *et al.*, 1983). At first sight, this strategy also appears to be unsuccessful: We have seen that there is no consistent evidence from correlational studies in this case either. However, if this strategy is applied in a different manner, described in the next section, it does indeed appear to be successful.

Manuck *et al.* (1989) observed that the area of laboratory-field research is beset by conceptual, methodological, and statistical difficulties. All of these factors may contribute to the differing results reported from correlational studies. In the next section we shall look at studies that employed the technique of multiple regression to examine relationships between laboratory reactivity and ambulatory mean levels of cardiovascular activity. These studies represent a strategy that may be more suited to this area of research. First, they conceptualize laboratory reactivity as one of several useful predictors that can be used together to predict ambulatory levels, as opposed to conceptualizing it as the sole predictor. Second, the technique of multiple regression allows the statistical implementation of this conceptualization.

Laboratory-Field Studies Employing Regression Analysis

This section describes three recent studies that employed regression analyses to explore the relationship between laboratory reactivity and ambulatory blood pressure levels. First, however, a brief explanation of the technique is appropriate.

The aim of multiple regression techniques is to predict an outcome (for example, ambulatory blood pressure levels) by using a combination of predictor variables. Each predictor variable is allowed to stay in the regression model being developed only if it contributes independent predictive power. This predictive power of an individual variable is usually expressed in terms of how much of the overall intersubject variance (100%) in ambulatory levels can be accounted for by that particular predictor variable. K. C. Light (1992, personal communication) has recommended the following strategy.

When trying to predict a person's real-world or ambulatory blood pressure levels, knowledge of his or her baseline (resting) blood pressure is particularly helpful. This item is therefore a main component of the regression model that is constructed. Knowledge of the subject's age is also informative. It is then appropriate to take into account several other measures known to influence blood pressure. To do so, complete and detailed behavioral diary information is needed, emphasizing the importance of these diaries. If this information is available, it is possible to take into account the influences of posture, recent exercise, emotional stress, social interactions, and caffeine and nicotine exposure. Other approaches may involve using measures of chronic life stress (such as working conditions, low socioeconomic status, low social support, and high perceived life stress scores) for measures of emotional stress.

These variables (or an appropriate subset of them) can be added sequentially to baseline blood pressure in a multiple predictor model. Those which improve the model, by accounting for new portions of the overall variance, are then retained while those which do not are deleted. Once all this has been done, we are in a position to test the hypothesis of interest to us, which is: Does knowledge of people's laboratory reactivity scores improve prediction of their ambulatory blood pressure levels?

To test this hypothesis, reactivity measures are added as the final predictor variables tested in these regression models. This tells us whether knowledge of reactivity scores contributes new predictive power *over and above* knowledge of all the other influences that are affecting blood pressure. This strategy allows a reasonable test of laboratory reactivity's contribution to ambulatory blood pressure, after both evaluating and controlling for the influence of other important variables known to influence blood pressure (K. C. Light, 1992, personal communication).

Having seen how the technique of multiple regression can be employed in investigations of laboratory-field associations, we can examine three recent studies that used this strategy. The first, by Ironson and colleagues (Ironson *et al.*, 1989), employed four laboratory tasks (a video game, bicycle exercise, the cold pressor, and the Type A Structured Interview) in addition to an ambulatory monitoring phase. Regression analyses determined that reactivity to the structured interview added significantly to the prediction of ambulatory blood pressure levels over and above the use of baseline values as predictors. An extra 3% to 7% of the variance in ambulatory data was accounted for by the inclusion of reactivity information.

The second study, by Ewart and Kolodner (1993), also employed ambulatory monitoring and four laboratory tasks; these included a

video game, mental arithmetic, mirror drawing, and a social competence interview. The social competence interview (see also Ewart &
Kolodner, 1991) is "a semi-structured interview designed to measure
subjects' propensity to experience recurring cardiovascular arousal
related to their personal goals, social skills, problem-solving strategies,
and interpersonal resources" (Ewart & Kolodner, 1993, p. 32). The
subject population on this occasion consisted of adolescents, and the
ambulatory monitoring phase occurred during school hours. Regression analyses revealed that reactivity to the social competence interview
added significantly to the prediction of ambulatory pressure over and
above the predictive power of baseline information. An extra 3% to 10%
of ambulatory variance was explained by use of these reactivity scores.

The social competence interview used in this study warrants further mention. Most of the reactivity tasks discussed in this book, with
the notable exception of speech tasks, have been nonsocial cognitive or
perceptual-motor tasks. Ewart and colleagues have suggested that the
use of this task may provide information not revealed by the use of
nonsocial tasks. Because interpersonal challenges arise often in daily
life, tasks that include some aspect of social challenge (e.g., public
speaking, role playing, and interviews) may elicit the cognitive, emotional and behavioral patterns that are likely to prevail in daily life
(Ewart & Kolodner, 1991, 1993). These authors suggest that such tasks be
included along with other reactivity tasks in a battery of stressors.

The third study, by Light and colleagues (Light *et al.*, 1993b),
measured blood pressure and hemodynamic responses during five
laboratory stressors. Subjects also completed a phase of ambulatory
blood pressure monitoring during work hours. Regression analyses
revealed that various reactivity measures added significantly to the
prediction of ambulatory pressures over and above the use of a "base"
regression model that incorporated information about baseline pressures, age, and posture. In this study, 4% to 13% of additional ambulatory pressure variance was explained by the addition of reactivity
information into the regression model.

These three studies yielded very similar results. While baseline
values account for large amounts of variance in ambulatory data,
reactivity to laboratory tasks can seemingly be used to contribute extra
predictive power. It is true to say that the amount of extra variance
explained by reactivity (which was remarkably similar in these studies)
is not overwhelming, but it is very important to recognize that this
addition in explained variance is a significant contribution that should

not be minimized. When trying to predict ambulatory values from laboratory data, each and every contribution is to be welcomed.

These studies conceptualize the role of reactivity in predicting ambulatory pressures in a manner different from correlational studies. Correlational studies explore the predictive power of reactivity by itself. In contrast, multiple regression models conceptualize reactivity as one of several predictors, knowledge of all of which is required to predict ambulatory pressures successfully. As Light and colleagues (Light et al., 1993b) commented, the differences between people in overall ambulatory pressures are the result of many constitutional factors (such as age, gender, body size, obesity, physical fitness level) and many environmental factors (posture, physical activity, smoking, eating, drinking) in addition to any reactivity that may occur as a result of mental activity and exposure to stress. Furthermore, the influence of many of these other factors is relatively prolonged, whereas reactivity exerts its influence only during relatively short, intermittent periods.

It is therefore hardly surprising that reactivity by itself is not always able to explain individual differences in mean levels of ambulatory blood pressure. However, if it is assumed that many constitutional influences are reflected in the *baseline* level of blood pressure, it becomes quite logical to employ a regression strategy in which baseline values are used as the initial predictor, and the potential predictive power of reactivity is assessed by evaluating the degree to which the addition of reactivity information *improves* the prediction of ambulatory levels (Light et al., 1993b).

Two other recent studies also employed regression strategies to examine aspects of laboratory-field generalization. In one, van Doornen and van Blokland (1992) used regression analysis to explore relationships between laboratory reactivity and a specific real-world stressor, namely, the public defense of a doctoral thesis. Laboratory reactivity scores added significantly to the prediction of ambulatory pressures over and above prediction on the basis of baseline values. Second, Gellman and colleagues (Gellman et al., 1990) used regression analysis to examine the influences of posture, place, and mood on ambulatory blood pressure. Posture was found to be a major determinant of ambulatory pressures. After controlling for posture, significant place and mood effects were found when subjects were sitting but not when they were standing (Gellman et al., 1990). Again, multivariate regression techniques allowed different important influences to be examined together, and the influence of the less powerful ones (place and mood) to be examined after evaluating and controlling for the most powerful one (posture).

Postural and Hemodynamic Considerations

When moving from the tight experimental control of the experimental psychophysiological laboratory into the domain of real-world ambulatory monitoring, one encounters a whole new set of methodological problems. However, ambulatory information is extremely important, and it will undoubtedly be used increasingly in future studies (Manuck et al., 1989; Pickering, 1989). This means that more attention will very likely be focused on dealing with the problems caused by extraneous influences such as proximity to meals, physical activity, and postural adjustments (see also Van Egeren, 1992). Physical activity, for example, has a large influence on cardiovascular activity. Researchers are therefore devising methods of measuring concomitant physical activity and then statistically removing variations in the data arising from variations in physical activity (e.g., Anastasiades & Johnston, 1990; Johnston et al., 1990).

With regard to postural influences, it has also become recognized that these, too, must be both examined and accounted for. The section below discusses a study that examined postural influences on both cardiovascular activity at rest and cardiovascular reactivity to a psychological stressor. While ultimate interest lies with postural influences in real-world situations, these influences were examined on this occasion in the laboratory. The experimental control possible in the laboratory allowed postural influences to be examined on this occasion in the absence of other extraneous influences present in real-world settings.

Postural Effects on Cardiovascular Activity

It is widely documented that posture affects resting blood pressure. Typically, blood pressures in three positions have been examined: lying, sitting, and standing. We shall focus on the seated and standing positions since these are the positions in which most real-world stressors are likely to be encountered. While almost instantaneous cardiovascular changes occur when changing posture, steady levels of activity are soon achieved in both the seated and standing positions (e.g., Rushmer, 1976; Turjanmaa, 1989). Compared with seated levels, mean systolic pressure levels will be little different when standing, while mean diastolic levels will be somewhat higher.[1] It should be noted, however, that while this information about mean pressures is widely available, there is much less information published concerning *individual differences* in blood pressure alterations from one posture to another. Individual differences in cardiovascular activity are extremely important in this research field. Accordingly, Turner and Sherwood (1991) examined these individual differences, as well as examining reactivity in both postures.

Twenty subjects provided baseline data in both postures, and also completed a mental arithmetic task in both postures.[2] Table 9.2 presents data addressing the first aspect of the study. Baseline blood pressures (both systolic and diastolic) are presented for each posture. Also shown is the change from one posture to the other; these change scores are calculated as "standing baseline minus seated baseline." The mean change scores are very much in line with expectations derived from the literature. On average, standing systolic pressure was 3.9 mmHg *lower* than when seated, whereas diastolic pressure was 8.6 mmHg *higher* when standing. However, hidden behind these mean values is enormous individual variation. For systolic pressure, the range in changes in pressure was from a *decrease* of 18.5 mmHg to an *increase* of 13.0 mmHg. For diastolic pressure, while there were no decreases, the increases in pressure ranged from zero to 17.5 mmHg.

Turning to the second aspect of the study, reactivity scores for each

---

[1]Some studies have found mean standing *systolic* pressure to be slightly lower than seated levels (Turjanmaa, 1989; Turner & Sherwood, 1991), and others have found it to be slightly higher (Hunt *et al.*, 1989; Sparrow *et al.*, 1986). This difference between studies may be attributable to differences in precise methodologies, and also to the exact nature of subject samples. Given the considerable individual differences in postural adjustment that are discussed in the text, the mean postural adjustment will depend on those selected as subjects. In contrast, mean *diastolic* pressure was found in each of the four studies mentioned here to be several millimeters of mercury higher in the standing position.

[2]In this study, subjects actually completed two task sessions in each posture. Correlational analysis revealed significant similarity between sessions (see Chapter 5), which was of particular interest for the standing task sessions since a standing task had not been reported in this manner before. Subsequently, data were averaged across the pairs of sessions in each posture to yield one task score for each posture (a procedure discussed in Chapter 7).

Table 9.2. Individual Systolic and Diastolic Pressure Baselines in Each
Posture, and the Change between Postures (20 subjects)

	Systolic (mmHg)			Diastolic (mmHg)		
	Seated	Standing	Change	Seated	Standing	Change
Subject						
1	127.0	108.5	−18.5	73.0	75.0	+2.0
2	129.5	113.0	−16.5	78.0	79.5	+1.5
3	128.0	112.5	−15.5	64.5	70.0	+5.5
4	126.0	110.5	−15.5	71.0	71.0	0.0
5	116.5	107.5	−9.0	70.5	79.5	+9.0
6	128.5	119.5	−9.0	70.0	81.0	+11.0
7	142.5	135.0	−7.5	80.5	82.5	+2.0
8	118.0	111.0	−7.0	66.0	71.5	+5.5
9	121.5	115.5	−6.0	63.0	75.0	+12.0
10	120.0	118.0	−2.0	64.5	81.0	+16.5
11	131.0	129.0	−2.0	76.0	84.0	+8.0
12	128.0	126.5	−1.5	71.0	82.0	+11.0
13	137.0	136.0	−1.0	75.0	84.5	+9.5
14	123.5	123.5	0.0	71.0	83.5	+12.5
15	115.0	116.5	+1.5	60.5	60.5	0.0
16	109.0	112.0	+3.0	63.0	77.0	+14.0
17	106.0	109.0	+3.0	58.5	76.0	+17.5
18	127.0	132.5	+5.5	65.5	76.0	+10.5
19	116.0	122.0	+6.0	68.0	81.0	+13.0
20	118.0	131.0	+13.0	73.5	85.0	+11.5
Mean values	123.4	119.5	−3.9	69.2	77.8	+8.6

posture were calculated by subtracting the respective baseline (either
the seated or the standing baseline) from the task level in that posture.
Correlation coefficients were calculated comparing seated reactivity
with standing reactivity. Blood pressure reactivity scores in the two
postures were *not* significantly associated with each other (r (18) = 0.27
and 0.42 for systolic and diastolic pressures, respectively). In other
words, responses to *exactly the same task* completed in different postures
were not significantly related to each other. Given this finding, perhaps
it is not surprising that a lack of association is often found between
blood pressure responses to a laboratory stressor completed while
seated and to a *different* stressor met in the real world while standing.

The Future Use of Ambulatory Hemodynamic Variables

Currently, ambulatory monitors can provide ambulatory heart rate and blood pressure data, but the technology for ambulatory hemodynamic assessment is not yet commercially available. However, this situation may well change before too long, and the use of ambulatory impedance cardiography may provide such data. This type of data may be particularly interesting in the context of laboratory-field generalization (Sherwood, 1993).

To illustrate this possibility, some further data collected in the posture study discussed in the previous section can be used. In addition to measuring blood pressure, cardiac output and total peripheral resistance data were also collected (Sherwood & Turner, 1993). Reactivity scores to the mental arithmetic task were calculated for both of these variables for each of the two postures. Unlike the blood pressure responses themselves, the responses of these underlying hemodynamic responses *were significantly associated* in the different postures. The correlation coefficients were 0.85 ($p < 0.0001$) for cardiac output and 0.65 ($p < 0.005$) for total peripheral resistance.

These results show that an individual whose blood pressure responses tend to be mediated primarily via cardiac output increases in one posture will tend to display blood pressure responses mediated in the same way in the second posture. Exactly the same is true for other individuals whose blood pressure responses tend to be mediated primarily via vascular (peripheral resistance) influences. Because it is very possible that, during a day's ambulatory monitoring, stressors will be encountered in both the seated and the standing positions, the use of hemodynamic variables may prove to be particularly illuminating when laboratory data are compared with data collected during ambulatory monitoring.

Summary

In this chapter we have examined the relationship between laboratory cardiovascular measures and those taken in the real world via ambulatory monitoring. Knowledge of people's cardiovascular activity in their natural environments is very important. If cardiovascular responses to stress play any role in the development of disease, it is these everyday responses that will be responsible.

Research in this area suggests that there is not an easily revealed relationship between laboratory reactivity and ambulatory pressures. Knowledge of reactivity by itself is not always a successful predictor of real-world blood pressure activity. However, it appears that reactivity can be quite useful as one of several items used to predict these real-world pressures.

Our present knowledge of laboratory-field generalization is less than perfect, and the precise nature of many real-world modulating factors (e.g., interpersonal interactions, social support, occupational responsibilities) needs further investigation (Turner & Sherwood, 1991). However, as our laboratory-field investigative techniques become more sophisticated, and as our knowledge of these modulating factors increases, our understanding of laboratory-field associations will, it is hoped, improve commensurately.

Further Reading

1. Fredrikson, M., Robson, A., & Ljungdell, T. (1991). Ambulatory and laboratory blood pressure in individuals with negative and positive family history of hypertension. *Health Psychology*, *10*, 371–377.
2. Fredrikson, M., Tuomisto, M., Lundberg, U., & Melin, B. (1990). Blood pressure in healthy men and women under laboratory and naturalistic conditions. *Journal of Psychosomatic Research*, *34*, 675–686.
3. Harshfield, G.A., James, G.D., Schlussel, Y., Yee, L.S., Blank, S.G., & Pickering, T.G. (1988). Do laboratory tests of blood pressure reactivity predict blood pressure changes during everyday life? *American Journal of Hypertension*, *1*, 168–174.
4. Langewitz, W., Ruddel, H., Schachinger, H., & Schmieder, R. (1989). Standardized stress testing in the cardiovascular laboratory: Has it any bearing on ambulatory blood pressure values? *Journal of Hypertension*, *7* (Suppl. 3), 41–48.
5. Light, K.C., Turner, J.R., Hinderliter, A., & Sherwood, A. (1993). Race and gender comparisons: II. Predictions of work blood pressure from laboratory baseline and cardiovascular reactivity measures. *Health Psychology*, *12*, 366–375.
6. McKinney, M.E., Miner, M.H., Ruddel, H., McIlvain, H.E., Witte, H., Buell, J.C., Eliot, R.S., & Grant, L.B. (1985). The standardized mental stress test protocol: Test-retest reliability and comparison with ambulatory blood pressure monitoring. *Psychophysiology*, *22*, 453–463.
7. Parati, G., Pomidossi, G., Albini, F., Malaspina, D., & Mancia, G. (1987). Relationship of 24-hour blood pressure mean and variability to severity of target-organ damage in hypertension. *Journal of Hypertension*, *5*, 93–98.
8. Turner, J.R., Ward, M.M., Gellman, M.D., Johnston, D.W., Light, K.C., & van Doornen, L.J.P. (1993). The relationship between laboratory and ambulatory cardio-

vascular activity: Current evidence and future directions. *Annals of Behavioral Medicine*, in press.

9. Van Doornen, L.J.P., & van Blokland, R.W. (1992). The relationship between cardiovascular and catecholamine reactions to laboratory and real-life stress. *Psychophysiology, 29*, 173–181.

10. Van Egeran, L.F., & Gellman, M.D. (1992). Cardiovascular reactivity to everyday events. In E.H. Johnson, W.D. Gentry, & S. Julius (Eds.), *Personality, elevated blood pressure, and hypertension* (pp. 135–150). Washington, DC: Hemisphere.

CHAPTER **10**

The Risk Identification Protocol

In this chapter we shall attempt to stand back and take a broader look at the phenomenon of reactivity, how best to evaluate it, and possible connections to hypertensive disease. The preceding chapters have addressed specific aspects in our examination of cardiovascular response to psychological stress in detail, and so reiteration will be avoided as much as possible. Instead, this chapter speculates on the possible application of reactivity testing in the cardiovascular risk ascertainment process.

Risk Prediction

The precise role of reactivity in the hypertensive etiological process is not known at this time; future research, it is hoped, will further our knowledge in this regard. However, for present purposes, we do not require this detailed knowledge. Regardless of whether reactivity is a mechanism, a marker, or a modifier (see Lovallo & Wilson, 1992a; Manuck *et al.*, 1990), we need to consider how best to evaluate it, and how to determine whether reactivity is a useful *predictor* of future pathophysiology. If the occurrence of high reactivity at a young age is shown reliably to predict future disease states, this is a very useful fact regardless of whether or not it leads *directly* to that endpoint. The mode of intervention may very well depend on the answer to the "mechanism, marker, or modifier" question, but the need for intervention of some kind does not.

A currently prevalent view in reactivity research (reflected throughout this volume) is that if there is a connection between reactivity and hypertension, it is consistently high reactivity in an individual that will be predictive of disease. However, at this stage it might be advisable to acknowledge that other characteristic reactivity patterns, such as extreme *instability*, may be indicative of pathophysiology (J. A. McCubbin, personal communication, 1992). It should be noted that the risk identification protocol presented in this chapter advocates repeated testing using multiple stressors, thus allowing the identification of various characteristic reactivity patterns that may eventually prove to be indicative of later disease.

Assessing reactivity is just one aspect of assessing cardiovascular disease risk. The overall risk ascertainment process requires that many factors be considered, and we shall look at this process shortly. First, however, the most appropriate way of assessing an individual's characteristic reactivity will be considered. Several authors have recently addressed this topic (e.g., Kamarck *et al.*, 1992; Manuck *et al.*, 1990; Pickering & Gerin, 1990; Sherwood & Turner, 1992), and readers are referred to their work on this topic for more detailed considerations.

Ewart and Kolodner (1991) have compared the process of reactivity assessment to that of the psychometric assessment of other behavioral traits (cardiovascular reactivity itself can be considered a behavioral trait, referring to an individual's propensity to exhibit an alteration in cardiovascular activity when faced with an eliciting stimulus). They have likened different reactivity tasks to items on a scale, with each item (task) contributing distinct information about the underlying construct (reactivity). Reactivity assessment using a diverse battery of stressors therefore seems a particularly useful approach.

What kinds of tasks should be included in such a battery? Standardized cognitive tasks, containing the element of standardized flexibility discussed in Chapter 3, seem appropriate (see Kamarck *et al.*, 1992). Standardized tasks eliciting blood pressure responses primarily via different mechanisms (cardiac output or total peripheral resistance alterations) may be informative; tasks such as the cold-pressor task might therefore be employed. Tasks involving some element of harassment (see Suarez & Williams, 1989) might be useful, as might speech tasks and physical exercise tasks, both dynamic and isometric (see Goble & Schieken, 1991). The Social Competence Interview (Ewart & Kolodner, 1991) discussed in the previous chapter, and other interview tasks, might prove very informative. Ambulatory monitoring should also be part of our overall assessment package. It also seems highly advisable, if not crucial, to test people more than once.

There is an argument, which in many ways seems plausible, that the tasks we choose should reflect the situations we face in everyday life; that is, they should have ecological validity. Some of the esoteric tasks employed in our research laboratories do not appear to have a lot of ecological validity, and this is of concern in some contexts. In the context of the present chapter, however, a different viewpoint is pertinent. If a task (any task) proves to be a reliable indicator of disease risk, then that task is useful. The evolutionary reasons for neural wiring to be sensitive to mental arithmetic, for example, are not completely clear. Nonetheless, if responses to such a task prove to be useful predictors, then the task should not be dismissed on ideological grounds alone. It is possible (though admittedly unlikely, but the point is still valid) that cardiovascular responses to a new task, such as standing on our heads and reciting the alphabet backwards, may prove to be the strongest predictor of disease yet found. If this is so, this task should be used even if we never perform anything remotely similar in our everyday lives.

The Risk Identification Protocol

Figure 10.1 presents a Risk Identification Protocol, which suggests the type of information that may prove useful in the risk ascertainment process. The first part of this protocol, the Cardiovascular Response File, shows the information that might be gathered during the application of a standardized battery of stressors. Resting data (or baseline data) obtained in more than one position (recall the discussion of posture in Chapter 9; see also Turner & Sherwood, 1991) are included along with reactivity data from both psychological and physical stressors (see also Jorde & Williams, 1986). The concept of physical stress testing has become widely accepted (e.g., following cardiac events as part of rehabilitation programs), but the concept of the routine application of mental stress testing is not yet so accepted. However, this may prove to be a very useful part of the overall risk assessment strategy. At this time, individual tasks are not shown. We have already considered several potentially useful tasks, and others may be found in due course. The most important point here is probably that we should use several different tasks.

Recovery data should also be collected. Rate of recovery following task cessation is used routinely in physical stress testing (for example,

Figure 10.1. The Risk Identification Protocol. The two files within this protocol, the Cardiovascular Response File and the Biopsychosocial File, suggest the kinds of information that might be used to establish an overall index of risk for cardiovascular disease.

Cardiovascular Response File

Task

Responses

	HR	SBP	DBP	CO	TPR	Other Parameters
Session # ___						
Resting Status						
Seated						
Standing						
Mental Stress Testing						
Task 1						
Recovery						
Task 2						
Recovery						
Task n						
Recovery						

Physical Stress Testing						
Task 1						
Recovery						
Task 2						
Recovery						
Task n						
Recovery						
Temporal Stability Evaluation						
Intertask Consistency Evaluation						
Ambulatory Data, Day #____						
Average Levels						
Home/Work/Sleep						
Variability						
Home/Work/Sleep						
Response to Identified Stressors						
Home/Work						

(continued)

Figure 10.1. (Continued)

Biopsychosocial File

Item	Information
Aerobic Fitness Level Exercise habits	
Blood-tested Factors Cholesterol, etc.	
Dietary Habits Alcohol Caffeine Smoking pattern	
Parental Cardiovascular Status Mother Father	
Personality Characteristics Hostility	

Renal Adequacy

Size
    Body Mass Index
    Height
    Weight

Social Support Assessment
    Home and work information
    Number of close friends
    Contacts per unit time

Typical Day Profile
    Domestic situation
    Job stress exposure
    "Job strain" index
    Habitual life stressors

as one index of physical fitness), and it may prove to be very informative in the context of mental stress testing (recall the Light *et al.* [1993a] study discussed in Chapter 8). Some of the physiological parameters that might usefully be measured are shown; but, again, this list is not meant to be definitive or exhaustive.

The second part of the Risk Identification Protocol is called the Biopsychosocial File. Apart from obtaining reactivity data, the risk ascertainment process requires obtaining additional information. Once we are able to define individuals as high reactors, it is possible that only a subset of this group will go on to develop hypertension (see Lovallo & Wilson, 1992a). Therefore, knowledge of reactivity status alone may not be enough to guarantee successful risk prediction (see DeQuattro & Lee, 1991). Accordingly, it is appropriate to gather all potentially useful information. The Biopsychosocial File collects information about a variety of relevant factors. Again, the contents of this file are meant to be neither definitive nor exhaustive. Instead, they simply show the type of information that may be helpful to collect.

Some of the items in this file need little explanation since they are routinely assessed already (e.g., parental history of cardiovascular disease, and body size). Some of these factors can operate in conjunction with each other. For example, children with initially high levels of blood pressure are more likely to become hypertensive adults, particularly if they are obese as children or become obese as young adults, and if they have a family history of hypertension (Mahoney *et al.*, 1991). However, other items in this file are not yet routinely assessed, although they may prove informative. Social support is a concept that is currently receiving a lot of attention (e.g., see Cohen & Syme, 1985; Monroe, 1989; Shumaker & Czajkowski, 1992; Strogatz & James, 1986). Evidence indicates that longevity increases with social support (House *et al.*, 1988), and laboratory work has suggested that social support may decrease reactivity (Gerin *et al.*, 1992; Kamarck *et al.*, 1990; see also Smith *et al.*, 1989; Smith *et al.*, 1990).

"Job strain" has also received recent attention. Job strain has been defined as the combination of high psychological demands together with low decision-making latitude at work (Karasek *et al.*, 1988). Current evidence suggests that high job strain is associated with higher ambulatory blood pressure at work in men but not in women (Light *et al.*, 1992c; Schnall *et al.*, 1990).

Various questionnaires may also provide useful information here. Examples are the Multiple Affect Adjective Check List (Revised) for measures of anxiety and hostility (Zuckerman & Lubin, 1985), the Daily Stress Inventory (Brantley *et al.*, 1988), the State-Trait Anger Scale (Spielberger *et al.*, 1983), the Life Situation Survey (Chubon, 1987), the Manifest Anxiety Scale (Bendig, 1956; see also Jamner *et al.*, 1988; Weinberger *et al.*, 1979), the Revised Ways of Coping Checklist (see Vitaliano *et al.*, 1993; see also Folkman & Lazarus, 1980), the Self-Concealment Scale (Larson & Chastain, 1990), the Social Desirability Scale (Crowne & Marlowe, 1964), the Social Readjustment Rating Scale and Schedule of Recent Events (Holmes & Rahe, 1967), and the Spielberger Anger Expression Scale (Spielberger *et al.*, 1985).

When it comes to calculating an overall score for both files, it may be the case that certain weightings should be applied to individual items. One particular item's occurrence may be particularly significant, and therefore this item should influence the overall average more strongly than items less powerful in their predictive ability. Eventually, all items may carry an individual weighting that is directly proportional to their predictive significance. It is also possible, however, that risk factors may combine with each other in an interactive nature, rather than an additive nature. The joint occurrence of two items that individually are not too significant may increase the overall risk considerably. A prediction-indexed weighting system may therefore need careful construction. One way to help construct such a weighting system is via appropriately designed follow-up studies.

Long-Term Follow-up Studies

The best way to determine the predictive powers of individual items contained in the Risk Identification Protocol, and the predictive powers of a combined index of these items, is to conduct appropriate prospective studies. Thorough evaluation needs to occur in young subjects, and then these subjects need to be followed for a considerable period of time. While this goal obviously requires considerable investment of time and energy, the information provided should make this investment well worthwhile.

Before looking briefly at the form such prospective studies might take, it is appropriate here to review some of the prospective studies already completed. Relatively few such studies have yet been reported. These were recently discussed by Light *et al.* (1992b), and the reader is referred to their review for a more detailed examination.

The cold pressor task has been used in prospective research in this area since the 1930s. Hines (1940) reported a 6-year follow-up of 66 individuals, all normotensive at the initial time of testing. During the 6-year interval none of the low reactors (to the cold pressor) developed hypertension, while one-third of the high reactors did so. While some subsequent studies (e.g., Armstrong & Rafferty, 1950; Harlan *et al.*, 1964) failed to replicate such a finding, more recent studies have brought renewed interest to the cold pressor as a potential predictor of hypertension.

A particularly noteworthy study is that of Menkes *et al.* (1989). This study has arguably provided the most powerful demonstration of the predictive power of reactivity to date, owing in part to its large sample size, its excellent retrieval rate on follow-up, and its long follow-up interval (Light *et al.*, 1992b). Results indicated that subjects whose systolic pressure reactivity to the cold pressor placed them in the top quarter of reactors had a greater incidence of hypertension from age 40 onwards compared to the less reactive subjects. In addition, when the effects of standard risk factors such as resting systolic blood pressure, family history of hypertension, age, height-weight index, and cigarette smoking were statistically removed, the risk associated with high systolic reactivity remained significant.

Other research scientists have employed mental, or psychological, stressors in prospective studies. Mental effort is indeed a prevalent component of contemporary life, and therefore experimental tasks that attempt to elicit the responses that real-life stressors may evoke may prove informative in long-term follow-up studies. Falkner and her colleagues (Falkner *et al.*, 1981) employed a mental arithmetic task in a study employing normotensive and borderline hypertensive adolescents. The borderline hypertensive group was more reactive to the mental arithmetic task than was the normotensive group at initial testing. Also, the subjects in the borderline hypertensive group who became hypertensive (the "hypertensive" group) were those who had shown the greatest reactivity during the mental arithmetic task. However, while this study indicates an association between high reactivity and hypertension development, it does not show that reactivity is an independent predictor of hypertension development. There were also group differences in parental history of hypertension as well as in reactivity.

Borghi *et al.* (1986) also employed a mental arithmetic task to test 44 young adults who initially had borderline hypertension. At follow-up 5 years later, nine subjects had developed essential hypertension. All of these subjects had initially demonstrated hyperreactivity during the mental arithmetic task. Of the remaining 35 subjects who did not display essential hypertension at follow-up, only 21% had shown large magnitude reactivity 5 years earlier. Interestingly, those subjects who went on to develop hypertension did *not* differ from the other subjects in their resting blood pressure levels. These results indicate that blood pressure reactivity is an independent predictor of later hypertension development. However, it was not a perfect predictor, since some subjects who showed high reactivity did not go on to develop hypertension. Almost certainly, other factors need to be assessed in addition to reactivity (hence the comprehensiveness of the Risk Identification Protocol).

Another study of interest here was recently reported by Light *et al.*, 1992a). This study represented a 10- to 15-year prospective follow-up of 51 initially healthy nonhypertensive individuals who had undergone reactivity testing as college students. The fact that these subjects were normotensive at the time of testing was in contrast to the borderline hypertensive status of the subjects in the Borghi *et al.* (1986) study noted earlier. Because borderline hypertension itself is a predictor of later essential hypertension, the assessment of the independent predictive power of reactivity in that study was somewhat compromised. Results of the study by Light and colleagues indicated that subjects with above-average heart rate reactivity during a reaction time task exhibited higher systolic and diastolic pressure than did less reactive men under several conditions (stethoscopic assessment, and work, social and leisure conditions) at follow-up. The authors commented that this study indicated that high cardiovascular reactivity "is at minimum a marker for later blood pressure elevations," but also noted that future research is needed to try to determine whether high reactivity is not just a marker for, but also plays a causal role in, the development of hypertension (Light *et al.*, 1992a).

There is now a general consensus that long-term prospective studies are very much needed in this area (e.g., see Fredrikson & Matthews, 1990; Manuck *et al.*, 1990; Matthews *et al.*, 1986b). What form might these studies take? First, the initial reactivity assessments should be comprehensive, along the lines suggested in the Risk Identification Protocol's Cardiovascular Response File. Second, the initial testing should take place while subjects are young, preferably before age 25 (Light *et al.*, 1992b). Third, a long follow-up interval is needed; Light *et al.* (1992b) suggested the goal of a mean follow-up duration of 25 to 30 years at minimum. Finally, comprehensive information pertaining to the individual's life (along the lines suggested by the Biopsychosocial File) should be gathered throughout the follow-up interval. In this manner, the independent predictive powers of individual items, and combinations of items, might be determined. This determination could perhaps be achieved by the use of the multiple regression techniques discussed in the previous chapter.

Summary

Reactivity testing may well be a useful component in the cardio-vascular risk ascertainment process. The Risk Identification Protocol presented in this chapter suggests the type of information that might usefully be collected. The protocol contains two files, the Cardiovascular Response File and the Biopsychosocial File. The first file shows the kinds of information that could be gathered during the application of a standardized battery of stressors. It is important to use different types of stressors (both mental and physical tasks), to collect baseline, task, and recovery data, and to administer the tasks more than once.

The Biopsychosocial File contains other items of potential relevance to cardiovascular disease. These include aerobic fitness level, dietary habits, parental history data, personality characteristics, and several other items. Not all high reactors may go on to develop hypertension. Therefore, since knowledge of reactivity status alone may not guarantee successful risk prediction, the additional information from the second file is likely to be quite useful.

To determine the predictive powers of items in the Risk Identification Protocol, long-term follow-up studies are needed. Following thorough evaluation at an early age, subjects need to be followed for a considerable time. When this has been done, multiple regression techniques appear well-suited to determine the independent predictive powers of individual items within the files, and of combinations of these items.

Further Reading

1. Borghi, C., Costa, F., Boschi, S., Mussi, A., & Ambrosioni, E. (1986). Predictors of stable hypertension in young borderline subjects: A five-year follow-up study. *Journal of Cardiovascular Pharmacology, 8* (Suppl. 5), S138–S141.

2. Ewart, C.K., & Kolodner, K.B. (1991). Social competence interview for assessing physiological reactivity in adolescents. *Psychosomatic Medicine, 53*, 289–304.

3. Falkner, B., Kushner, H., Onesti, G., & Angelakos, E.T. (1981). Cardiovascular characteristics in adolescents who develop essential hypertension. *Hypertension, 3*, 521–527.

4. Fredrikson, M., & Matthews, K.A. (1990). Cardiovascular responses to behavioral stress and hypertension: A meta-analytic review. *Annals of Behavioral Medicine, 12*, 30–39.

5. Kamarck, T.W., Manuck, S.B., & Jennings, J.R. (1990). Social support reduces cardiovascular reactivity to psychological challenge: A laboratory model. *Psychosomatic Medicine, 52*, 42–58.

6. Kamarck, T.W., Jennings, J.R., Debski, T.T., Glickman-Weiss, E., Johnson, P.S., Eddy, M.J., & Manuck, S.B. (1992). Reliable measures of behaviorally-evoked cardiovascular reactivity from a PC-based test battery: Results from student and community samples. *Psychophysiology, 29*, 17–28.

7. Light, K.C., Dolan, C.A., Davis, M.R., & Sherwood, A. (1992). Cardiovascular responses to an active coping challenge as predictors of blood pressure patterns 10 to 15 years later. *Psychosomatic Medicine, 54*, 217–230.

8. Light, K.C., Sherwood, A., & Turner, J.R. (1992). High cardiovascular reactivity to stress: A predictor of later hypertension development. In J.R. Turner, A. Sherwood, & K.C. Light (Eds.), *Individual differences in cardiovascular response to stress* (pp. 281–293). New York: Plenum.

9. Lovallo, W.R., & Wilson, M.F. (1992). A biobehavioral model of hypertension development. In J.R. Turner, A. Sherwood, & K.C. Light (Eds.), *Individual differences in cardiovascular response to stress* (pp. 265–280). New York: Plenum.

10. Menkes, M.S., Matthews, K.A., Krantz, D.S., Lundberg, V., Mead, L.A., Qaqish, B., Liang, K.-Y., Thomas, C.B., & Pearson, T.A. (1989). Cardiovascular reactivity to the cold pressor test as a predictor of hypertension. *Hypertension, 14*, 524–530.

CHAPTER 11

Other Areas of Cardiovascular
Reactivity and Behavioral Medicine
Research and Some Final Thoughts

This volume has addressed the use of the psychophysiological strategy in the investigation of how cardiovascular reactivity might be related to the development of essential hypertension. As indicated in Chapter 1, we have focused on the first part of Schwartz and Weiss's (1978, p. 250) definition of behavioral medicine, that is, on "the development and integration of behavioral and biomedical science knowledge and techniques relevant to health and illness." At this point in the text, however, it is appropriate to mention some of the areas of reactivity research that have not been discussed in detail, and to provide the reader with some further readings that can serve as a starting point for following up on topics of particular interest.

Other Research Topics

Assessment of Catecholamines in Reactivity Studies

One topic that has received no direct attention in this book is the assessment of catecholamines in stress research. Blood levels of the catecholamines (particularly epinephrine and norepinephrine) are a potentially valuable guide to sympathetic nervous system activity (Ziegler, 1989). Many laboratory studies similar in nature to those presented in this volume have evaluated catecholamine responses during stress. Indeed, while those results were not discussed, some of the studies included in this text also monitored catecholamine activity as well as cardiac activity. Readers are referred to the work of Ziegler and colleagues (e.g., Dimsdale & Ziegler, 1991; Ziegler, 1989; Ziegler et al., 1991) and Frankenhaeuser and colleagues (see Frankenhaeuser, 1991) for information concerning the employment of catecholamines in stress research.

Coronary Heart Disease

Although research findings on both hypertension and coronary heart disease share some common ground, coronary heart disease is also a major avenue of investigation in its own right. Endpoints such as angina pectoris, atherosclerosis, myocardial ischemia, and myocardial infarction have received considerable attention in the literature (e.g., Bosimini et al., 1991; Dembroski & Costa, 1988; Haynes & Matthews, 1988; Perkins, 1989; Schneiderman et al., 1989; Steptoe,1981). For a particularly readable introduction to coronary heart disease, the reader is referred to Smith and Leon (1992).

Various Topics

Other topics of interest include the relationship between caffeine consumption and reactivity (Lane et al., 1990; Shapiro et al., 1986), the renin-angiotensin-aldosterone system (Atlas et al., 1989), endogenous opioids (McCubbin et al., 1992), other potential markers of sympathetic nervous system activity such as chromogranin A and neuropeptide Y (Mills & Dimsdale, 1992), silent ischemia (Norvell et al., 1989), adrenergic receptors (Girdler et al., 1992; Mills & Dimsdale, 1988, 1993; Sherwood & Hinderliter, 1993), platelet aggregation (Grignani et al., 1991; Markovitz & Matthews, 1991), serum lipid concentrations (Waldstein et al., 1993), and the use of nonhuman primates as a model for evaluating behavioral influences on cardiovascular structure and function (Kaplan et al., 1991; McCubbin et al., 1993; Manuck et al., 1986).

Attention has also focused on left ventricular mass index. Left ventricular hypertrophy is the thickening of the wall of the ventricle. This condition, along with abnormal left ventricular diastolic function, is an important end-organ manifestation of hypertension that contributes significantly to the morbidity and mortality associated with this cardiovascular disease (Hinderliter et al., 1991).

Finally, several recent studies have explored the relationship between cardiovascular reactivity and immune function (see the readings listed in the Psychoneuroimmunology section of this chapter's Further Reading). High reactors have been shown to demonstrate greater immunological change than low reactors, with low reactors showing little or no change (see Kiecolt-Glaser *et al.*, 1992). Such studies suggest a convergence of cardiovascular, neuroendocrine, and psychoneuroimmunological research and the evaluation of differences among individuals who vary in autonomic activation (Kiecolt-Glaser *et al.*, 1992). This convergence may be helpful in identifying individuals predisposed to long-term health changes.

Examples of papers addressing other areas are provided at the end of this chapter. These topics, which by no means comprise an exhaustive list, serve to illustrate the richness and diversity of individual lines of inquiry within contemporary cardiovascular behavioral medicine and psychosomatic medicine research.

Intervention Strategies

If and when it is decided unequivocally that large magnitude reactivity has deleterious cardiovascular consequences, our attention must focus in a concentrated manner on ways in which such reactivity might be eliminated, or (perhaps more realistically) significantly reduced. There has already been research conducted on several modes of intervention, and it is appropriate to consider some examples briefly at this point.

First, however, it should be noted that intervention can basically take two forms: pharmacological and behavioral. As we discover more about the mechanisms underlying blood pressure responses in certain situations, and about how certain individuals' responses are mediated primarily by one mechanism while those of other individuals are primarily mediated by a different one, various pharmacological agents may become widely employed. (See Mills & Dimsdale, 1991; Shapiro *et al.*, 1986; Surwit, 1986, for reviews of pharmacological agents as modulators of reactivity.) Although pharmacological intervention is currently extremely important in treating cardiovascular disease, in keeping with the theme of this volume, we are presently more interested in behavioral interventions.

Such interest is also in line with the observation of Kaufmann, Chesney, and Weiss (1991) that the greatest impact on public health can be achieved through changes in behavior. While the damage inflicted through certain maladaptive behaviors such as substance abuse, smoking, and inappropriate eating patterns is clear, it is also possible, if harder to demonstrate, that behavioral factors are involved in the etiology of hypertension.

Reactivity

We shall consider four strategies that have been used to explore the possible modification of reactivity to psychological and psychosocial stressors: aerobic exercise, social support, biofeedback, and relaxation. Laboratory reactivity has been reduced by each strategy.

As was noted in Chapter 8, the effects of single bouts of exercise on physiological responses immediately following the exercise have been studied. Roy and Steptoe (1991) found that systolic, diastolic, and heart rate responses to mental arithmetic in male subjects were significantly attenuated following a 20-minute period of high-level exercise on a bicycle ergometer. As a second example here, Rejeski et al. (1992) investigated the effects of a demanding 40-minute bout of bicycle exercise on women's blood pressure reactivity during the Stroop word-matching task and a public-speaking task. Again, exercise was seen to dampen blood pressure reactivity. (See also Pescatello et al., 1991.)

Second, consider laboratory models of social support. Good social support appears to be protective with regard to cardiovascular morbidity and mortality (see House et al., 1988). Kamarck et al. (1990) employed a paradigm in which subjects received support in the form of the presence of a friend while they completed two laboratory stressors (mental arithmetic and a concept-formation task). Blood pressure and heart rate reactivity were reduced by social support relative to an experimental condition in which subjects performed the tasks alone.

Gerin et al. (1992) also examined the possibility that social support may operate as a moderator of cardiovascular reactivity. In this study, the task was a psychosocial stressor in which subjects were the object of verbal attack in a discussion of a controversial issue (abortion, euthanasia, the death penalty, or gun control). In the "social support" condition, a "supportive" individual (a confederate of the experimenters) provided agreement with the subject. In the "no support" condition, a "neutral" individual sat passively throughout the discussion and provided no support. Subjects in the social support condition showed significantly less cardiovascular reactivity than did subjects in the no-support condition.

Third, Larkin and colleagues have investigated the use of biofeed-back in the regulation of heart rate during a video game task (Larkin *et al.*, 1989, 1990, 1992a, 1992b). In one of these studies (Larkin *et al.*, 1990), each subject participated in a pretraining assessment of cardiovascular reactivity, a training condition, and a posttraining assessment identical to the initial evaluation. There were four training conditions: (1) a habituation control group; (2) an instruction-only control group (who received instructions to maintain a low or unchanged heart rate during the task); (3) a feedback group that received instructions to lower heart rate using ongoing heart rate feedback; and (4) a feedback group receiving instructions to lower heart rate, and given heart rate feedback plus a score contingency in which participants' total game score was jointly determined by their game performance and their success at heart rate control.

Results showed that subjects in both feedback conditions exhibited greater reductions in heart rate reactivity during the posttraining video-game assessment than did subjects in both control groups. The greatest reductions were shown by the subjects who received feedback and the score contingency.

Finally, McCubbin's group recently completed a study examining the effects of relaxation training on cardiovascular reactivity (J. A. McCubbin, personal communication, 1993). Jacobsonian progressive muscular relaxation training (Jacobson, 1938) was employed. Twenty-eight young adult males with mildly elevated resting blood pressure were randomly assigned, either to a group receiving relaxation training, or to a nontraining control group. Cardiovascular measures were taken both before and after the training/control intervention condition while subjects performed a 10-minute computer-operated mental arithmetic task. Relative to nontraining controls, subjects in the relaxation training group exhibited significantly reduced diastolic blood pressure reactivity.

Hypertension

Behavioral interventions that may be useful in the case of hyperten-sion include relaxation therapy, meditation, stress management, bio-feedback, control of diet, weight loss, physical exercise, and cognitive therapy (learning to view a situation that was previously considered stressful in a new, nonstressful manner). However, the clinical evidence for the benefits of behavioral interventions to date is, at best, inconsistent (for a review of the effects of relaxation therapy, see Jacob *et al.*, 1991; for weight management, see Jeffery, 1991; for exercise, see Siegel & Blumenthal, 1991; for biofeedback, meditation, and cognitive therapy, see Jacob & Chesney, 1986).

However, we should not be discouraged. Rather, given the considerable potential benefit of nonpharmacological interventions, we should redouble our efforts and consider why this inconsistent picture exists in the literature. Two possibilities suggest themselves. First, as Kaufmann *et al.* (1991) noted, it may be that the behavioral interventions employed to date are not sufficiently relevant to the physiology of hypertension. Second, it may be the case that our employment of available strategies, and our evaluation of their effects, has not been sophisticated enough; perhaps we as behavioral medicine practitioners need to implement the intervention strategies in a better way. Treatment schedules must be designed and implemented that include consideration of habits and lifestyle, development of dietary and exercise programs, and the development of requisite levels of commitment and motivation (Kaufmann *et al.*, 1991).

Stress Management Programs

Stress management can be defined as "any behavioural or psychological procedure offered or undertaken that deliberately attempts to alter beneficially any aspect of the stress process, including altering the environment, subjective appraisal of that environment, and the subjective, behavioural and physiological responses to the stressful experience" (Johnston, 1992, p. 58). Stress management has been used for both hypertension and coronary heart disease, and there is some evidence that it can lead to a reduction in cardiovascular disease (see Johnston, 1989, 1992). However, considerable future research is needed here.

Although this book focuses on cardiovascular concerns, chronic life stress can lead to poor health evidenced in a number of body systems. For example, ulcers, migraine headaches, and immunological function may all have stress-related components. Greenberg (1993) provides examples of the many different types of life stressors we encounter. These include (1) environmental stressors (toxins, heat, cold); (2) psychological stressors (threats to self-esteem, depression); (3)

sociological stressors (unemployment, death of a loved one); and (4) philosophical stressors (use of time, purpose in life). In his introduction to the topic of comprehensive stress management, Greenberg (1993) focuses on psychological and sociological stressors and introduces techniques such as perception interventions, meditation, relaxation, and strategies for decreasing stressful behaviors. Readers are also referred to the volume edited by Lehrer and Woolfolk (1993), which provides a detailed account of the theory and practice of stress management.

The "Opening Your Heart" Program

Based on his pioneering research published in the *Lancet* and other leading medical journals, Dr. Dean Ornish has developed the Opening Your Heart program. His research has demonstrated that it is possible to *reverse* coronary heart disease by making changes in life-style—that is, without using pharmacological or surgical interventions (Ornish, 1990). These life-style changes can also help to prevent heart disease.

Life-style factors can activate all mechanisms known to cause coronary heart disease and heart attacks (Ornish, 1990). Given this observation, it is appropriate to pay attention to diet, consumption of nicotine and stimulants, exercise, and emotional stress. To prevent coronary artery disease, or to help reverse it if it is already present, Ornish advocates a low-fat vegetarian diet, regular exercise, and "opening your heart to your feelings and to inner peace." A major theme of his book states that "treating only the physical manifestations of heart disease without addressing the more fundamental causes will provide only temporary relief, and the disease is likely to recur. At best, we will trade one set of problems for another" (Ornish, 1990, p. 27). Techniques to decrease isolation (from our inner self and inner peace, from others, and from a higher force) and increase intimacy are described and advocated. The program therefore pays attention to physical, emotional, and spiritual aspects of opening, and healing, one's heart.

Again, it should be noted here that Ornish's book does not minimize the benefits of medication and surgery. Both of these are important. The program described by Ornish should be considered an adjunct to, not a substitute for, conventional medical therapy (Ornish, 1990).

Stress Inoculation Training

Stress inoculation training originated in the discipline of clinical psychology, and it is a form of cognitive-behavioral therapy. Rather than being a single technique, stress inoculation training is "a generic term referring to a treatment paradigm consisting of a semistructured, clinically sensitive training regimen" (Meichenbaum, 1985, p. 21). Analogous in some ways to medical inoculations, this training is designed to enhance resistance to psychological stressors through exposure to stimuli that are strong enough to arouse defenses without being so powerful that they overcome them (Meichenbaum, 1985).

Stress inoculation training can be carried out with individuals, couples, and with groups. It consists of many elements including teaching, discussion, cognitive restructuring, problem solving and relaxation training, and behavioral and imaginal rehearsal. Three main phases of the training are called the *conceptualization phase, skills acquisition and rehearsal*, and *application and follow-through*.

Stress inoculation training has been applied in many settings, including public-speaking anxiety, fear of flying, and preparation for open heart surgery. It can also be useful with regard to stress at work. In addition to nurturing coping skills in individual clients, environmental modifications and job redesign can be encouraged, via cooperation between workers and management, which can make the workplace less stressful. (See Meichenbaum, 1985, for further details and references.)

Some Final Thoughts

At this point it seems appropriate to stand back and try to obtain an overarching perspective on the material that we have covered in the previous chapters. The focus of this book has been to provide an introductory examination of the use of the psychophysiological experimental strategy to investigate cardiovascular reactivity within a behavioral medicine/psychosomatic medicine perspective. To do this, the relationship between reactivity and the development of hypertension has been employed as an example. Preceding chapters have examined specific areas in some detail. While that level of analysis is absolutely necessary, this final chapter aims for a more global view.

Presently, unequivocal evidence of the role of reactivity in the development of hypertension has not been provided. Certainly, some suggestive evidence has been presented, and plausible inferential arguments have been advanced, but categorical demonstration of such a link has not yet been offered. What does this lead us to conclude about the future of reactivity research? There are two main ways of looking at this situation. One view is that reactivity research may have little to offer (Pickering & Gerin, 1990, 1992). The second salient viewpoint here is that reactivity may indeed be connected with hypertension, but our behavioral science research techniques have so far been either inappropriate or not sufficiently sophisticated enough to be able to demonstrate this link.

Manuck *et al.* (1990, p. 27) suggested it is possible "that cardiovascular reactivity is still poorly understood as a construct of individual differences, and therefore is imperfectly assessed (or conceptualized) in its relationship to hypertension." These authors were encouraged by the observation that, even with the methodological and conceptual limitations of our still-developing discipline, available studies do suggest a possible association between heightened cardiovascular reactivity and hypertension. In encouraging future research, they suggested that such research should (1) use more comprehensive assessments of cardiovascular reactivity; (2) attempt to find out what factors underlie an enhanced cardiovascular responsivity (with particular attention directed toward central nervous system and peripheral mechanisms of relevance to hypertension); (3) address the question of causality in animal models; and (4) pursue models of association in human studies that encompass other attributes of risk germane to the multifactorial disorder of hypertension (Manuck *et al.*, 1990).

Future work on reactivity thus promises to provide interesting information. As Turner *et al.* (1992) noted, a complete understanding of biobehavioral interactions, and of any possible pathogenic consequences, requires that all useful avenues of inquiry and investigative techniques are combined appropriately in integrative research strategies. Such integrative strategies seem crucial in an area in which associations and interactions among different influences are so important. By considering the most recent advances in the conceptualization of relevant issues, the measurement techniques and experimental paradigms now available, and more sophisticated and promising analytical techniques, we may be able to reframe some of our questions so that we can better look for appropriate answers.

In addition to more sophisticated laboratory and field assessment of cardiovascular function and the use of human and nonhuman subjects, however, we must also employ other approaches. As Matthews observed, "the central questions in this area must ultimately be addressed by prospective, epidemiological studies of humans" (Matthews *et al.*, 1986b, p. 472). Admittedly, such studies are much more difficult to design and complete than are laboratory studies incorporating a small number of subjects. However, once done, the rewards will be commensurately greater. It will be interesting to follow the development of such studies.

As we refine our behavioral science skills, and accordingly conduct potentially more informative research, we must avoid one particular pitfall. While strict adherence to the medical model discourages consideration of psychological variables, psychologists and psychophysiologists must not commit the converse sin of omission by ignoring the physical (bodily) dimension. In all likelihood, any potentially deleterious psychological input will only affect susceptible biological programs, at least to any significant degree. Obrist (1981) encouraged us to become better biologists. In addition to continuing to refine our evaluations of behavioral impact, we also need to continue to study hypertension's "physiology and pharmacology" (Kaufmann *et al.*, 1991).

As regards an ultimate evaluation of the association between reactivity and hypertension, Popperian philosophy dictates that we must evaluate this hypothesis at some point in time; we cannot modify our theories indefinitely to account for all future observations. It is possible that reactivity may not be a cause of hypertension, a co-participant in the etiology of hypertension, or even a marker for risk conferred by other pathogenic factors, and it may not potentiate end-organ and vascular complications. If this is found to be the case, reactivity studies will contribute no clinically useful information (Manuck *et al.*, 1989). However, the author of this text would endorse suggestions (e.g., Manuck *et al.*, 1989) that the time for final evaluations of the reactivity hypothesis is not yet here. Readers who are currently students of cardiovascular psychophysiology, behavioral medicine, and psychosomatic medicine have the opportunity to address some fascinating questions in the coming years.

One goal of this volume has been to introduce in a self-contained fashion current cardiovascular reactivity research and future possibilities in the fields of cardiovascular behavioral medicine and psychosomatic medicine. Some topics have been discussed in considerable detail to provide a glimpse of the fundamentals of experimental research projects, while other chapters have provided a less detailed yet broader picture of related topics. A second goal has been to provide a starting point from which the reader may, if he or she chooses, pursue topics of particular interest. The reading lists at the end of each chapter, and the complete references at the end of the volume, should help here. Of course, each reference will itself contain more references, and the search for published knowledge can then occur as a precursor of further experimental investigation. Such investigation will be invaluable in illuminating the true nature of the hypothesized relationship between cardiovascular reactivity and cardiovascular disease.

Summary

Cardiovascular reactivity is one of several important topics within the field of cardiovascular behavioral medicine. Some of the others are the assessment of catecholamines in stress research, coronary heart disease, and intervention strategies. While these topics are not covered in detail, appropriate references have been provided to direct the reader who wishes to pursue them.

Reactivity research is strongly driven by the possibility of an association between reactivity and cardiovascular disease. Presently, no definitive evidence shows that reactivity is involved in the development of hypertension, but several experimental strategies do provide encouraging suggestive data. Further research is needed along several individual, but ultimately convergent, lines of inquiry.

Several forms of association between reactivity and hypertension may exist. It is possible that reactivity may be a cause of hypertension, a co-participant in the development of hypertension, or a noncausal marker for risk conferred by other pathogenic factors. More research, which takes full advantage of recent advances in conceptualization, methodological sophistication, and analytical strategies, is needed to explore each of these possibilities in greater detail. Such future investigation promises to be most illuminating.

Further Reading

In this chapter many additional readings are presented. They are divided into eight categories, but this classification system is far from definitive, and the categories are certainly not mutually exclusive. It is hoped that this system will help you find research areas of particular interest, and specific articles within those areas. Again, it is emphasized that this is by no means an exhaustive list; it is a starting point for your own further reading.

General Reading

Conference on behavioral medicine and cardiovascular disease. *Circulation* (Suppl.), P. 2, Vol. 76, No. 1, July 1987.
Gatchel, R.J., Baum, A., & Krantz, D.S. (1989). *An introduction to health psychology* (2nd ed.). New York: Random House.
Julius, S. (1991). Autonomic nervous system dysregulation in human hypertension. *American Journal of Cardiology, 67,* 3B–7B.
Julius, S. (1992). Relationship between the sympathetic tone and cardiovascular responsiveness in the course of hypertension. In E.H. Johnson, W.D. Gentry, & S. Julius (Eds.), *Personality, elevated blood pressure and essential hypertension* (pp. 219–230). Washington, DC: Hemisphere.
Krantz, D.S., & Manuck, S.B. (1984). Acute psychophysiologic reactivity and risk of cardiovascular disease: A review and methodologic critique. *Psychological Bulletin, 96,* 435–464.
Steptoe, A. (1991). Invited review: The links between stress and illness. *Journal of Psychosomatic Research, 35,* 633–644.
Steptoe, A., & Vögele, C. (1991). Methodology of mental stress testing in cardiovascular research. *Circulation, 83* (Suppl. II), II-14–II-24.

Ambulatory Monitoring

Anderson, D.E., Austin, J., & Haythornthwaite, J.A. (1993). Blood pressure during sustained inhibitory breathing in the natural environment. *Psychophysiology, 30,* 131–137.
Asmar, R.G., Girerd, X.J., Brahimi, M., Safavian, A., & Safar, M.E. (1992). Ambulatory blood pressure measurement, smoking and abnormalities of glucose and lipid metabolism in essential hypertension. *Journal of Hypertension, 10,* 181–187.
Berardi, L., Chau, N.P., Chanudet, X., Vilar, J., & Larroque, P. (1992). Ambulatory blood pressure monitoring: A critical review of the current methods to handle outliers. *Journal of Hypertension, 10,* 1243–1248.
Degaute, J-P., van de Borne, P., Kerkhofs, M., Dramix, M., & Linkowski, P. (1992). Does non-invasive ambulatory blood pressure monitoring disturb sleep? *Journal of Hypertension, 10,* 879–885.
Fredrikson, M., & Blumenthal, J.A. (1990). Serum lipid levels and ambulatory blood pressure. *Journal of Ambulatory Monitoring, 3,* 113–118.
Goldstein, I.B., Jamner, L.D., & Shapiro, D. (1992). Ambulatory blood pressure and heart rate in healthy male paramedics during a workday and a non-workday. *Health Psychology, 11,* 48–54.

Harshfield, G.A., Alpert, B.S., Willey, E.S., Somes, G.W., Murphy, J.K., & Dupaul, L.M. (1989). Race and gender influence ambulatory blood pressure patterns of adolescents. *Hypertension, 14*, 598–603.

Harshfield, G.A., Hwang, C., Blank, S.G., & Pickering, T.G. (1989). Research techniques for ambulatory blood pressure monitoring. In N. Schneiderman, S.M. Weiss, & P.G. Kaufmann (Eds.), *Handbook of research methods in cardiovascular behavioral medicine* (pp. 293–309). New York: Plenum.

Harshfield, G.A., Alpert, B.S., Pulliam, D.A., Willey, E.S., Somes, G.W., & Stapleton, F.B. (1991). Sodium excretion and racial differences in ambulatory blood pressure patterns. *Hypertension, 18*, 813–818.

Harshfield, G.A., Pulliam, D.A., Alpert, B.S., Stapleton, F.B., Willey, E.S., & Somes, G.W. (1991). Renin-sodium profiles influence ambulatory blood pressure patterns in children and adolescents. *Pediatrics, 87*, 94–100.

Imholz, B.P.M., Langewouters, G.J., van Montfrans, G.A., Parati, G., van Goudoever, J., Wesseling, K.H., Wieling, W., & Mancia, G. (1993). Feasibility of ambulatory, continuous 24-hour finger arterial pressure recording. *Hypertension, 21*, 65–73.

James, G.D. (1991). Race and perceived stress independently affect the diurnal variation of blood pressure in women. *American Journal of Hypertension, 4*, 382–384.

Jamner, L.D., Shapiro, D., Goldstein, I.B., & Hug, R. (1991). Ambulatory blood pressure and heart rate in paramedics: Effects of cynical hostility and defensiveness. *Psychosomatic Medicine, 53*, 393–406.

Krantz, D.S., Grabbay, F.H., Hedges, S.M., Leach, S.G., Gottdiener, J.S., & Rozanski, A. (1993). Mental and physical triggers of silent myocardial ischemia: Ambulatory studies using self-monitoring diary methodology. *Annals of Behavioral Medicine, 15*, 33–40.

Light, K.C., Turner, J.R., & Hinderliter, A.L. (1992). Job strain and ambulatory blood pressure in healthy young men and women. *Hypertension, 20*, 214–218.

Llabre, M.M., Ironson, G., Spitzer, S., Gellman, M., Weidler, D., & Schneiderman, N. (1988). Blood pressure stability of normotensive and mild hypertensive subjects in different settings. *Health Psychology, 7*, 127–137.

Mancia, G. (1990). Ambulatory blood pressure monitoring: Research and clinical applications. *Journal of Hypertension, 8* (Suppl. 7), S1–S13.

Matthews, K.A., Owens, J.F., Allen, M.T., & Stoney, C.M. (1992). Do cardiovascular responses to laboratory stress relate to ambulatory blood pressure levels?: Yes, in some of the people, some of the time. *Psychosomatic Medicine, 54*, 686–697.

Perloff, D., Sokolov, M., Cowan, R.M., & Juster, R.P. (1989). Prognostic value of ambulatory measurements: Further analyses. *Journal of Hypertension, 7* (Suppl. 3), S3–S10.

Pickering, T.G. (1992). The ninth Sir George Pickering memorial lecture: Ambulatory monitoring and the definition of hypertension. *Journal of Hypertension, 10*, 401–409.

Pickering, T.G. (1993). Applications of ambulatory blood pressure monitoring in behavioral medicine. *Annals of Behavioral Medicine, 15*, 26–32.

Pieper, C., Warren, K., & Pickering, T.G. (1993). A comparison of ambulatory blood pressure and heart rate at home and work on work and non-work days. *Journal of Hypertension, 11*, 177–183.

Pollak, M.H. (1991). Heart rate reactivity to laboratory tasks and ambulatory heart rate in daily life. *Psychosomatic Medicine, 53*, 25–35.

Sausen, K.P., Lovallo, W.R., Pincomb, G.A., & Wilson, M.F. (1992). Cardiovascular responses to occupational stress in male medical students: A paradigm for ambulatory monitoring studies. *Health Psychology, 11,* 55–60.

Schwan, A., & Eriksson, G. (1992). Effect on sleep—but not on blood pressure—of nocturnal non-invasive blood pressure monitoring. *Journal of Hypertension, 10,* 189–194.

Schwartz, G.L., Turner, S.T., & Sing, C.F. (1992). Twenty-four-hour blood pressure profiles in normotensive sons of hypertensive parents. *Hypertension, 20,* 834–840.

Spitzer, S.B., Llabre, M.M., Ironson, G.H., Gellman, M.D., & Schneiderman, N. (1992). The influence of social situations on ambulatory blood pressure. *Psychosomatic Medicine, 54,* 79–86.

Staessen, J.A., Fagard, R.H., Lijnen, P.J., Thijs, L., Hoof, R.V., & Amery, A.K. (1991). Mean and range of the ambulatory pressure in normotensive subjects from a meta-analysis of 23 studies. *American Journal of Cardiology, 67,* 723–727.

Undén, A.-L., Orth-Gomér, K., & Elofsson, S. (1991). Cardiovascular effects of social support in the workplace: Twenty-four-hour ECG monitoring of men and women. *Psychosomatic Medicine, 53,* 50–60.

Ward, M.M., Turner, J.R., & Johnston, D.W. (1993). Temporal stability of cardiovascular ambulatory monitoring. *Annals of Behavioral Medicine,* in press.

White, W.B., Berson, A.S., Robbins, C., Jamieson, M.J., Prisant, M., Roccella, E., & Sheps, S.G. (1993). National standard for measurement of resting and ambulatory blood pressures with automated sphygmomanometers. *Hypertension, 21,* 504–509.

Coping Strategies

Cohen, S., & Syme, S.L. (1985). *Social support and health.* New York: Academic Press.

Dolan, C.A., & White, J.W. (1988). Issues of consistency and effectiveness in coping with daily stressors. *Journal of Research in Personality, 22,* 395–407.

Dolan, C.A., Sherwood, A., & Light, K.C. (1992). Cognitive coping strategies and blood pressure responses to real-life stress in healthy young men. *Health Psychology, 11,* 233–240.

Folkman, S., Lazarus, R.S., Dunkel-Schetter, C., DeLongis, A., & Gruen, R.J. (1986). The dynamics of a stressful encounter: Cognitive appraisal, coping and encounter outcomes. *Journal of Personality and Social Psychology, 50,* 992–1003.

King, A.C., Barr Taylor, C., Albright, C.A., & Haskell, W.L. (1990). The relationship between repressive and defensive coping styles and blood pressure responses in healthy, middle-aged men and women. *Journal of Psychosomatic Research, 34,* 461–471.

Krogh, V., Trevisan, M., Jossa, F., Bland, S., Jalowiec, A., Celentano, E., Farinaro, E., Panico, S., Fusco, G., & Mancini, M. (1992). Coping and blood pressure. *Journal of Human Hypertension, 6,* 65–70.

Lazarus, R.S., & Folkman, S. (1984). *Stress, appraisal and coping.* New York: Springer.

Niaura, R., Herbert, P.N., McMahon, N., & Sommerville, L. (1992). Repressive coping and blood lipids in men and women. *Psychosomatic Medicine, 54,* 698–706.

Parkes, K.R. (1986). Coping in stressful episodes: The role of individual differences, environmental factors and situational characteristics. *Journal of Personality and Social Psychology, 51,* 1277–1292.

Roth, S., & Cohen, L.J. (1986). Approach, avoidance and coping with stress. *American Psychologist, 41,* 813–819.

Steptoe, A. (1989). Coping and psychophysiological reactions. *Advances in Behavior Research Therapy*, 11, 259–270.

Steptoe, A., & Appels, A. (1989). *Stress, personal control and health*. Chichester: Wiley.

Stone, A.A., Neale, J.M., & Shiffman, S. (1993). Daily assessments of stress and coping and their association with mood. *Annals of Behavioral Medicine*, 15, 8–16.

Hypertension

Blaustein, M.P., & Hamlyn, J.M. (1991). Pathogenesis of essential hypertension.: A link between dietary salt and high blood pressure. *Hypertension*, 18 (Suppl. III), III-184–III-195.

Bohr, D.F., Dominiczak, A.F., & Webb, R.C. (1991). Pathophysiology of the vasculature in hypertension. *Hypertension*, 18 (Suppl. III), III-69–III-75.

Brandão, A.P., Brandão, A.A., Araújo, E.M., & Oliveira, R.C. (1992). Familial aggregation of arterial blood pressure and possible genetic influence. *Hypertension*, 19 (Suppl. II), II-214–II-217.

Brody, M.J., Varner, K.J., Vasquez, E.C., & Lewis, S.J. (1991). Central nervous system and the pathogenesis of hypertension: Sites and mechanisms. *Hypertension*, 18 (Suppl. III), III-7–III-12.

Brum, J.M., Tramposch, A.F., & Ferrario, C.M. (1991). Neurovascular mechanisms and sodium balance in the pathogenesis of hypertension. *Hypertension*, 17 (Suppl. I), I-45–I-51.

DiBona, G.F. (1991). Stress and sodium intake in neural control of renal functioning in hypertension. *Hypertension*, 17 (Suppl. III), III-2–III-6.

DiBona, G.F. (1992). Sympathetic neural control of the kidney in hypertension. *Hypertension*, 19 (Suppl. I), I-28–I-35.

DiBona, G.F., & Jones, S.Y. (1992). Arterial baroreceptor reflex function in borderline hypertensive rats. *Hypertension*, 19, 56–61.

Ferrannini, E. (1992). The haemodynamics of obesity: A theoretical analysis. *Journal of Hypertension*, 10, 1417–1423.

Floras, J.S. (1992). Epinephrine and the genesis of hypertension. *Hypertension*, 19, 1–18.

Frohlich, E.D. (1991). The heart in hypertension: A 1991 overview. *Hypertension*, 18 (Suppl. III), III-62–III-68.

Gans, R.O., & Donker, A.J. (1991). Insulin and blood pressure regulation. *Journal of Internal Medicine* (Suppl.), 735, 49–64.

Gillman, M.W., Oliveria, S.A., Moore, L.L., & Ellison, R.C. (1992). Inverse association of dietary calcium with systolic blood pressure in young children. *Journal of the American Medical Association*, 267, 2340–2343.

Guyton, A.C. (1991). Abnormal renal function and autoregulation in essential hypertension. *Hypertension*, 18 (Suppl. III), III-49–III-53.

Hall, J.E., Brands, M.W., Hildebrant, D.A., & Mizelle, H.L. (1992). Obesity-associated hypertension: Hyperinsulinemia and renal mechanisms. *Hypertension*, 19 (Suppl. I), I-45–I-54.

Hansson, L. (1991). Review of state-of-the-art beta-blocker therapy. *American Journal of Cardiology*, 67, 43B–46B.

Jern, S., Bergbrant, A., Bjorntorp, P., & Hansson, L. (1992). Relation of central hemodynamics to obesity and body fat distribution. *Hypertension*, 19, 520–527.

McCubbin, J.A., Kaufmann, P.G., & Nemeroff, C.B. (1991). *Stress, neuropeptides, and systemic disease*. Orlando, FL: Academic Press.

Mathias, C.J. (1991). Management of hypertension by reduction in sympathetic activity. *Hypertension, 17* (Suppl. III), III-69–III-74.

Pickering, T.G., Devereux, R.B., Gerin, W., James, G.D., Pieper, C., Schlussel, Y.R., & Schnall, P.L. (1990). The role of behavioral factors in white coat and sustained hypertension. *Journal of Hypertension* (Suppl.), *8*, S141–S147.

Pickering, T.G., Schnall, P.L., Schwartz, J.E., & Pieper, C.F. (1991). Can behavioral factors produce a sustained elevation of blood pressure? Some observations and a hypothesis. *Journal of Hypertension* (Suppl. 8), *9*, S66–S68.

Skyler, J.S., Donahue, R.P., Marks, J.B., Thompson, N.E., & Schneiderman, N. (1992). Insulin: A determinant of blood pressure? In E.H. Johnson, W.D. Gentry, & S. Julius (Eds.), *Personality, elevated blood pressure, and essential hypertension* (pp. 257–281). Washington, DC: Hemisphere.

Sleight, P. (1991). Role of the baroreceptor reflexes in circulatory control, with particular reference to hypertension. *Hypertension, 18* (Suppl. III), III-31–III-34.

Sullivan, J.M. (1991). Salt sensitivity: Definition, conception, methodology and long-term issues. *Hypertension, 17* (Suppl. I), I-61–I-68.

Tuck, M.L. (1992). Obesity, the sympathetic nervous system and essential hypertension. *Hypertension, 19* (Suppl. I), I-67–I-77.

Intervention Strategies

Achmon, J., Granek, M., Golomb, M., & Hart, J. (1989). Behavioral treatment of essential hypertension: A comparison between cognitive therapy and biofeedback of heart rate. *Psychosomatic Medicine, 51*, 152–164.

Beech, H.G., Burns, L.E., & Sheffield, B.F. (1982). *A behavioural approach to the management of stress*. Chichester: Wiley.

Bennett, P., Wallace, L., Carroll, D., & Smith, N. (1991). Treating type A behaviours and mild hypertension in middle-aged men. *Journal of Psychosomatic Research, 35*, 209–223.

Cohen, S., & Syme, L.S. (1985). *Social support and health*. New York: Academic Press.

Frasure-Smith, N., & Prince, R. (1989). Long-term follow-up of the Ischemic Heart Disease Life Stress Monitoring Program. *Psychosomatic Medicine, 51*, 485–513.

Goleman, D.J., & Schwartz, G.E. (1976). Meditation as an intervention in stress reactivity. *Journal of Consulting and Clinical Psychology, 44*, 456–466.

Greenberg, J.S. (1993). *Comprehensive stress management*. Dubuque, IA: Wm. C. Brown.

Heber, M.E., Broadhurst, P.A., Brigden, G.S., & Raftery, E.B. (1990). Effectiveness of the once-daily calcium antagonist, lacidipine, in controlling 24-hour ambulatory blood pressure. *American Journal of Cardiology, 66*, 1228–1232.

Hypertension Prevention Trial Research Group. (1990). The hypertension prevention trial: Three-year effects of dietary changes in blood pressure. *Archives of Internal Medicine, 150*, 153–162.

Jacob, R.G., & Chesney, M.A. (1986). Psychological and behavioral methods to reduce cardiovascular reactivity. In K.A. Matthews, S.M. Weiss, T. Detre, T.M. Dembroski, B. Falkner, S.B. Manuck, & R.B. Williams, Jr. (Eds.), *Handbook of stress, reactivity and cardiovascular disease* (pp. 417–457). New York: Wiley.

Jacob, R.G., Shapiro, A.P., O'Hara, P., Portser, S., Kruger, A., Gatsonis, C., & Ding, Y. (1992). Relaxation therapy for hypertension: Setting-specific effects. *Psychosomatic Medicine, 54,* 87–101.

Johnston, D.W. (1989). Prevention of cardiovascular disease by psychological methods. *British Journal of Psychiatry, 154,* 183–194.

Johnston, D.W. (1991). Stress management in the treatment of mild primary hypertension. *Hypertension, 17 (Suppl. III),* III-63–III-68.

Johnston, D.W. (1992). The management of stress in the prevention of coronary heart disease. In S. Maes, H. Leventhal, & M. Johnston (Eds.), *International review of health psychology* (pp. 57–83). New York: Wiley.

Johnston, D.W., Gold A., Kentish, J., Smith, D., Vallance, P., Shah, D., Leach, G., & Robinson, B. (1993). The effects of stress management on blood pressure in mild primary hypertensives. *British Medical Journal, 306,* 963–966.

Kaufmann, P.G., Chesney, M.A., & Weiss, S.M. (1991). Behavioral medicine in hypertension: Time for new frontiers? *Annals of Behavioral Medicine, 13,* 3–4.

McGrady, A., Nadsady, P.A., & Schumann-Brzezinski, C. (1991). Sustained effects of biofeedback-assisted relaxation therapy in essential hypertension. *Biofeedback and Self-Regulation, 16,* 399–411.

Meichenbaum, D. (1985). *Stress inoculation training.* New York: Pergamon.

Norvell, N., & Belles, D. (1990). *Stress management training: A group leader's guide.* Sarasota, FL: Professional Resource Exchange.

Ornish, D., Brown, S.E., Scherwitz, L.W., Billings, J.H., Armstrong, W.T., Ports, T.A., McLanahan, S.M., Kirkeeide, R.L., Brand, R.J., & Gould, K.L. (1990). Can lifestyle change reverse coronary heart disease? *Lancet, 336,* 129–133.

Ornish, D., Scherwitz, L.W., Doody, R.S., Kesten, D., McLananhan, S.M., Brown, S.E., Depney, G., Sonnemaker, R., Haynes, C., Lester, J., McAllister, G.K., Hall, R.J., Burdine, J.A., & Gotto, A.M. (1983). Effects of stress management training and dietary change in treating ischemic heart disease. *Journal of the American Medical Association, 249,* 54–59.

Patel, C. (1975). Yoga and biofeedback in the management of "stress" in hypertensive patients. *Clinical Science and Molecular Medicine* (Suppl. 28), 171–174.

Patel, C., & Marmot, M.G. (1988). Can general practitioners use training in relaxation and management of stress to reduce mild hypertension? *British Medical Journal, 296,* 21–24.

Pickering, T.G. (1992). Predicting the response to nonpharmacologic treatment in mild hypertension. *Journal of the American Medical Association, 247,* 1256–1257.

Saab, P.G., Dembroski, T.M., & Schneiderman, N. (1992). Coronary-prone behaviors: Intervention issues. In K.D. Craig & S.M. Weiss (Eds.), *Health enhancement, disease prevention, and early intervention: Biobehavioral perspectives* (pp. 233–268). New York: Springer.

Siani, A., Strazzullo, P., Giacco, A., Pacioni, D., Celentano, E., & Mancini, M. (1991). Increasing dietary potassium intake reduces the need for antihypertensive medication. *Annals of Internal Medicine, 115,* 753–759.

The Trials of the Hypertension Prevention Collaborative Research Group. (1992). The effects of nonpharmacologic interventions on blood pressure of persons with high normal levels: Results of the trials of hypertension prevention, phase 1. *Journal of the American Medical Association, 267,* 1213–1220.

van Montfrans, G.A., Karemaker, J.M., Wieling, W., & Dunning, A.J. (1990). Relaxation therapy and continuous ambulatory blood pressure in mild hypertension: A controlled study. *British Medical Journal, 300,* 1368–1372.

Psychoneuroimmunology

Bachen, E.A., Manuck, S.B., Marsland, A.L., Cohen, S., Malkoff, S.B., Muldoon, M.F., & Rabin, B.S. (1992). Lymphocyte subset and cellular immune responses to a brief experimental stressor. *Psychosomatic Medicine, 54,* 673–679.

Dunn, A.J. (1989). Psychoneuroimmunology for the psychoneuroendocrinologist: A review of animal studies of nervous system–immune system interactions. *Psychoneuroendocrinology, 14,* 251–274.

Herbert, T.B., & Cohen, S. (1993). Stress and immunity in humans: A meta-analysis review. *Psychosomatic Medicine, 55,* 364–379.

Kiecolt-Glaser, J.K., & Glaser, R. (1990). Stress and immune function in humans. In R. Ader, D. Felten, & N. Cohen (Eds.), *Psychoneuroimmunology* (2nd ed.) (pp. 849–867). San Diego: Academic Press.

Kiecolt-Glaser, J.K., Cacioppo, J.T., Malarkey, W.B., & Glaser, R. (1992). Acute psychological stressors and short-term immune changes: What, why, for whom and to what extent? *Psychosomatic Medicine, 54,* 680–685.

Manuck, S.B., Cohen, S., Rabin, B.S., Muldoon, M.F., & Bachen, E.A. (1991). Individual differences in cellular immune responses to stress. *Psychological Science, 2,* 111–115.

Zakowski, S.G., McAllister, C.G., Deal, M., & Baum, A. (1992). Stress, reactivity and immune function in healthy men. *Health Psychology, 11,* 223–232.

Reactivity

Allen, M.T., & Crowell, M.D. (1990). The effects of paced respiration on cardiopulmonary responses to laboratory stressors. *Journal of Psychophysiology, 4,* 357–368.

Anderson, E.A., Mahoney, L.T., Lauer, R.M., & Clarke, W.R. (1987). Enhanced forearm blood flow during mental stress in children of hypertensive parents. *Hypertension, 10,* 544–549.

Brown, P.C., & Smith, T.W. (1992). Social influence, marriage, and the heart: Cardiovascular consequences of interpersonal control in husbands and wives. *Health Psychology, 11,* 88–96.

Christensen, A.J., & Smith, T.W. (1993). Cynical hostility and cardiovascular reactivity during self-disclosure. *Psychosomatic Medicine, 55,* 193–202.

Czajkowski, S.M., Hindelang, R.D., Dembroski, T.M., Mayerson, S.E., Parks, E.B., & Holl, J.C. (1990). Aerobic fitness, psychological characteristics and cardiovascular reactivity to stress. *Health Psychology, 9,* 676–692.

de Geus, E.J.C., van Doornen, L.J.P., & Orlebeke, J.F. (1993). Regular exercise and aerobic fitness in relation to psychological make-up and physiological stress reactivity. *Psychosomatic Medicine, 55,* 347–363.

de Geus, E.J.C., & van Doornen, L.J.P. (1993). The effects of training on the physiological stress-response. *Work and Stress,* in press.

Ditto, B., & Miller, S.B. (1989). Forearm blood flow responses of offspring of hypertensives to an extended stress task. *Hypertension, 13,* 181–187.

Engebretson, T.O., & Matthews, K.A. (1992). Dimensions of hostility in men, women and boys: Relationships to personality and cardiovascular responses to stress. *Psychosomatic Medicine, 54,* 311–323.

Engebretson, T.O., Matthews, K.A., & Scheier, M.F. (1989). Relations between anger expression and cardiovascular reactivity: Reconciling inconsistent findings through a matching hypothesis. *Journal of Personality and Social Psychology, 57,* 513–521.

Everson, S.A., Lovallo, W.R., Sausen, K.P., & Wilson, M.F. (1992). Hemodynamic characteristics of young men at risk for hypertension at rest and during laboratory stressors. *Health Psychology, 11,* 24–31.

Ewart, C.K., & Kolodner, K.B. (1992). Diminished pulse pressure to psychological stress: Early precursor of essential hypertension? *Psychosomatic Medicine, 54,* 436–446.

Falkner, B., & Kushner, H. (1991). Interaction of sodium sensitivity and stress in young adults. *Hypertension, 17* (Suppl. I), I-162–I-165.

France, C., & Ditto, B. (1992). Cardiovascular responses to the combination of caffeine and mental arithmetic, cold pressor and static exercise stressors. *Psychophysiology, 29,* 272–282.

Fredrikson, M., Tuomisto, M., & Bergman-Losman, B. (1991). Neuroendocrine and cardiovascular stress reactivity in middle-aged normotensive adults with parental history of cardiovascular disease. *Psychophysiology, 28,* 656–664.

Freedman, R.R., Sabharwal, S.C., & Desai, N. (1987). Sex differences in peripheral vascular adrenergic receptors. *Circulation Research, 61,* 581–585.

Gerin, W., Pieper, C., Marchese, L., & Pickering, T.G. (1992). The multi-dimensional nature of active coping: Differential effects of effort and enhanced control on cardiovascular reactivity. *Psychosomatic Medicine, 54,* 707–719.

Harbin, T.J. (1989). The relationship between the type A behavior pattern and physiological responsivity: A quantitative review. *Psychophysiology, 26,* 110–119.

Haythornthwaite, J.A., Pratley, R.E., & Anderson, D.E. (1992). Behavioral stress potentiates the blood pressure effects of a high sodium intake. *Psychosomatic Medicine, 54,* 231–239.

Houtman, I.L.D., & Bakker, F.C. (1991). Individual differences in reactivity to and coping with the stress of lecturing. *Journal of Psychosomatic Research, 35,* 11–24.

Hurwitz, B.E., Nelesen, R.A., Saab, P.G., Nagel, J.H., Spitzer, S.B., Gellman, M.D., McCabe, P.M., Phillips, D.J., & Schneiderman, N. (1993). Differential patterns of dynamic cardiovascular regulation as a function of task. *Biological Psychology, 36,* 75–95.

Jennings, J.R., Kamarck, T., Stewart, C., Eddy, M., & Johnson, P. (1992). Alternate cardiovascular baseline assessment techniques: Vanilla or resting baseline. *Psychophysiology, 29,* 742–750.

Johnson, E.H. (1989). Cardiovascular reactivity, emotional factors and home blood pressures in black males with and without a parental history of hypertension. *Psychosomatic Medicine, 51,* 390–403.

Johnson, E.H., Nazzaro, P., & Gilbert, D.C. (1991). Cardiovascular reactivity to stress in black male offspring of hypertensive parents. *Psychosomatic Medicine, 53,* 420–432.

Jorgensen, R.S., Nash, J.K., Lasser, N.L., Hymowitz, N., & Langer, A.W. (1988). Heart rate acceleration and its relationship to total serum cholesterol, triglycerides and blood pressure reactivity in men with mild hypertension. *Psychophysiology, 25,* 39–44.

Jorgensen, R.S., Gelling, P.D., & Kliner, L. (1992). Patterns of social desirability and anger in young men with a parental history of hypertension: Association with cardiovascular activity. *Health Psychology, 11,* 403–412.

Julius, S. (1988). The blood pressure seeking properties of the central nervous system. *Journal of Hypertension, 6,* 177–185.

Julius, S., Jones, K., Schork, N., Johnson, E., Krause, L., Nazzaro, P., & Zemva, A. (1991). Independence of pressure reactivity from pressure levels in Tecumseh, Michigan. *Hypertension, 17* (Suppl. III), III-12–III-21.

Kamarck, T.W. (1992). Recent developments in the study of cardiovascular reactivity: Contributions from psychometric theory and social psychology. *Psychophysiology, 29,* 491–503.

Kelsey, R.M. (1991). Electrodermal lability and myocardial reactivity to stress. *Psychophysiology, 28,* 619–631.

Kirschbaum, C., Wust, S., & Hellhammer, D. (1992). Consistent sex differences in cortisol responses to psychological stress. *Psychosomatic Medicine, 54,* 648–657.

Krantz, D.S., Helmers, K.F., Bairey, C.N., Nebel, L.E., Hedges, S.M., & Rozanski, A. (1991). Cardiovascular reactivity and mental stress-induced myocardial ischemia in patients with coronary artery disease. *Psychosomatic Medicine, 53,* 1–13.

Lai, J.Y., & Linden, W. (1992). Gender, anger expression style, and opportunity for anger release determine cardiovascular reaction to and recovery from anger provocation. *Psychosomatic Medicine, 54,* 297–310.

Lamensdorf, A.M., & Linden, W. (1992). Family history of hypertension and cardiovascular changes during high and low affect provocation. *Psychophysiology, 29,* 558–565.

Lane, J.D., & Manus, D.C. (1989). Persistent cardiovascular effects with repeated caffeine administration. *Psychosomatic Medicine, 51,* 373–380.

Light, K.C., & Turner, J.R. (1992). Stress-induced changes in the rate of sodium excretion in healthy black and white men. *Journal of Psychosomatic Research, 36,* 497–508.

Linden, W., & Frankish, J. (1988). Expectancy and type of activity: Effects on pre-stress cardiovascular adaptation. *Biological Psychology, 27,* 227–235.

Llabre, M.M., Ironson, G.H., Spitzer, S.B., Gellman, M.D., Weidler, D.J., & Schneiderman, N. (1988). How many blood pressure measures are enough? An application of generalizability theory to the study of blood pressure reliability. *Psychophysiology, 25,* 97–106.

McCubbin, J.A., Cheung, R., Montgomery, T.B., Bulbulian, R., & Wilson, J.F. (1992). Aerobic fitness and opioidergic inhibition of cardiovascular stress reactivity. *Psychophysiology, 29,* 687–697.

Manuck, S.B., Olsson, G., Hjemdahl, P., & Rehnqvist, N. (1992). Does cardiovascular reactivity to mental stress have prognostic value in postinfarction patients? A pilot study. *Psychosomatic Medicine, 54,* 102–108.

Matthews, K.A., Davis, M.C., Stoney, C.M., Owens, J.F., & Caggiula, A.R. (1991). Does the gender relevance of the stressor influence sex differences in psychophysiological responses? *Health Psychology, 10,* 112–120.

Miller, S.B. (1992). Affective moderators of the cardiovascular response to stress in offspring of hypertensives. *Journal of Psychosomatic Research, 36,* 149–157.

Miller, S.B. (1993). Cardiovascular reactivity in anger-defensive individuals: The influence of task demands. *Psychosomatic Medicine, 55,* 78–85.

Muldoon, M.F., Bachen, E.A., Manuck, S.B., Waldstein, S.R., Bricker, P.L., & Bennett, J.A. (1992). Acute cholesterol responses to mental stress and change in posture. *Archives of Internal Medicine, 152*, 775–780.

Murphy, J.K., Alpert, B.S., & Walker, S.S. (1992). Ethnicity, pressor reactivity and children's blood pressure: Five years of observations. *Hypertension, 20*, 327–332.

Nagel, J.H., Han, K., Hurwitz, B.E., & Schneiderman, N. (1992). Assessment and diagnostic applications of heart rate variability. *Biomedical Engineering-Applications, Basis and Communications, 4*, 1–8.

Rejeski, W.J., Thompson, A., Brubaker, P.H., & Miller, H.S. (1992). Acute exercise: Buffering psychosocial stress responses in women. *Health Psychology, 11*, 355–362.

Rozanski, A., Bairey, C.N., Krantz, D.S., Friedman, J., Resser, K.J., Morrell, M., Hilton-Chalfen, S., Hestrin, L., Bietendorf, J., & Berman, D.S. (1988). Mental stress and the induction of silent myocardial ischemia in patients with coronary artery disease. *New England Journal of Medicine, 318*, 1005–1012.

Saab, P.G., Tischenkel, N., Spitzer, S.B., Gellman, M.D., Pasin, R.D., & Schneiderman, N. (1991). Race and blood pressure status influences cardiovascular responses to challenge. *Journal of Hypertension, 9*, 249–258.

Siegman, A.W., Dembroski, T.M., & Crump, D. (1992). Speech rate, loudness and cardiovascular reactivity. *Journal of Behavioral Medicine, 15*, 519–532.

Sims, J., & Carroll, D. (1990). Cardiovascular and metabolic activity at rest and during psychological and physical challenge in normotensives and subjects with mildly elevated blood pressure. *Psychophysiology, 27*, 149–156.

Smith, T.W., & Brown, P. (1991). Cynical hostility, attempts to exert social control and cardiovascular reactivity in married couples. *Journal of Behavioral Medicine, 14*, 579–590.

Steptoe, A., Kearsley, N., & Walters, N. (1993). Cardiovascular activity during mental stress following vigorous exercise in sportsmen and inactive men. *Psychophysiology, 30*, 245–252.

Suarez, E.C., Williams, R.B., Jr., Kuhn, C.M., Zimmerman, E.H., & Schanberg, S.M. (1991). Biobehavioral basis of coronary-prone behavior in middle-aged men. Part II: Serum cholesterol, the type A behavior pattern and hostility as interactive modulators of physiological reactivity. *Psychosomatic Medicine, 53*, 528–537.

Thayer, J.F., van Doornen, L.J.P., & Turner, J.R. (1991). Calculation of additional heart rates using oxygen consumption and carbon dioxide production: A comparative analysis. *Behavior Research Methods, Instruments, and Computers, 23*, 2–4.

Tischenkel, N.J., Saab, P.G., Schneiderman, N., Nelesen, R.A., Pasin, R.D., Goldstein, D.A., Spitzer, S.B., Woo-Ming, R., & Weidler, D.J. (1989). Cardiovascular and neurohumoral responses to behavioral challenge as a function of race and sex. *Health Psychology, 8*, 503–525.

Vitaliano, P.P., Russo, J., Bailey, S.L., Young, H.M., & McCann, B.S. (1993). Psychosocial factors associated with cardiovascular reactivity in older adults. *Psychosomatic Medicine, 55*, 164–177.

Vögele, C., & Steptoe, A. (1992). Emotional coping and tonic blood pressure as determinants of cardiovascular responses to mental stress. *Journal of Hypertension, 10*, 1079–1087.

Ward, M.M., Swan, G.E., & Jack, L.M. (1993). Effect of smoking cessation and relapse on cardiovascular levels and reactivity. *Psychopharmacology*, in press.

Alternate Approaches to Cardiovascular Dynamics and Control

Berntson, G.G., Cacioppo, J.T., & Quigley, K.S. (1991). Autonomic determinism: The modes of autonomic control, the doctrine of autonomic space, and the laws of autonomic constraint. *Psychological Reviews, 98*, 459–487.

Friedman, B.H., Thayer, J.F., Borkovec, T.D., Tyrrell, R.A., Johnsen, B-H., & Colombo, R. (1993). Autonomic characteristics of nonclinical panic and blood phobia. *Biological Psychiatry, 34*, 298–310.

Goldberger, A.L. (1991). Is the normal heartbeat chaotic or homeostatic? *News in Physiological Science, 6*, 87–91.

Goldberger, A.L., & Rigney, D.R. (1990). Sudden death is not chaos. In S. Krasner (Ed.), *The ubiquity of chaos*. Washington, DC: American Association for the Advancement of Science.

Jennings, J.R. (1992). Is it important that the mind is in a body? Inhibition and the heart. *Psychophysiology, 29*, 369–383.

Jennings, J.R., van der Molen, M.W., Brock, K., & Somsen, R.J.M. (1991). Response inhibition initiates cardiac deceleration: Evidence from a sensory-motor compatibility paradigm. *Psychophysiology, 28*, 72–85.

Lombardi, F., Sandrone, G., Pernpruner, S., Sala, R., Garimoldi, M., Ceruti, S., Baseli, G., Pagani, M., & Malliani, A. (1989). Heart rate variability as an index of sympathovagal interaction after acute myocardial infarction. *American Journal of Cardiology, 60*, 1239–1245.

Malliani, A., Lombardi, F., Pagani, M., & Cerutti, S. (1990). Clinical exploration of the autonomic nervous system by means of electrocardiography. *Annals of the New York Academy of Science, 601*, 234–246.

Saul, J.P., (1990). Beat-to-beat variations of heart rate reflect modulation of cardiac autonomic outflow. *News in Physiological Science, 5*, 32–37.

References

Abel, J.L., & Larkin, K.T. (1991). Assessment of cardiovascular reactivity across laboratory and natural settings. *Journal of Psychosomatic Research, 35,* 365–373.

Ahlquist, R.P. (1976a). Adrenergic receptors in the cardiovascular system. In P.R. Saxena & R.P. Forsyth (Eds.), *Beta-adrenoceptor blocking agents* (pp. 29–34). Amsterdam: North Holland.

Ahlquist, R.P. (1976b). Present state of alpha and beta-adrenergic drugs: I. The adrenergic receptor. *American Heart Journal, 92,* 661–664.

Ahlquist, R.P. (1976c). Present state of alpha and beta-adrenergic drugs: II. The adrenergic blocking agents. *American Heart Journal, 92,* 804–807.

Allen, M.T., Sherwood, A., & Obrist, P.A. (1986). Interactions of respiratory and cardiovascular adjustments to behavioral stressors. *Psychophysiology, 23,* 532–541.

Allen, M.T., Sherwood, A., Obrist, P.A., Crowell, M.D., & Grange, L.A. (1987). Stability of cardiovascular reactivity to laboratory stressors: A 2½-year follow-up. *Journal of Psychosomatic Research, 31,* 639–645.

Alli, C., Avanzini, F., DiTullio, M., Mariotti, G., Salmoirago, E., Taioli, E., & Radice, M. (1990). Left ventricular diastolic function in normotensive adolescents with different genetic risk of hypertension. *Clinical Cardiology, 12,* 115–118.

Alpert, B.S., & Wilson, D.K. (1992). Stress reactivity in childhood and adolescence. In J.R. Turner, A. Sherwood, & K.C. Light (Eds.), *Individual differences in cardiovascular response to stress* (pp. 187–201). New York: Plenum.

Alpert, B.S., Somes, G.W., Harshfield, G.A., & Schieken, R.M. (1992, June). *Genetic influence on 24-hour blood pressure patterns.* Paper presented at the Seventh International Congress on Twin Studies: Tokyo, Japan.

Anastasiades, P., & Johnston, D.W. (1990). A simple activity measure for use with ambulatory subjects. *Psychophysiology, 27,* 87–93.

Anderson, D.E., Dietz, J.R., & Murphy, P. (1987). Behavioral hypertension in sodium-loaded dogs is accompanied by sustained sodium retention. *Journal of Hypertension, 5,* 99–105.

Anderson, D.E., Kearns, W.D., & Better, W.E. (1983). Progressive hypertension in dogs by avoidance conditioning and saline infusion. *Hypertension, 5,* 286–291.

Anderson, N.B. (1989). Ethnic differences in resting and stress-induced cardiovascular and humoral activity: An overview. In N. Schneiderman, S.M. Weiss, & P.G.

Kaufmann (Eds.), *Handbook of research methods in cardiovascular behavioral medicine* (pp. 433–451). New York: Plenum.

Anderson, N.B., McNeilly, M., & Myers, H. (1992). Toward understanding race differences in autonomic reactivity: A proposed contextual model. In J.R. Turner, A. Sherwood, & K.C. Light (Eds.), *Individual differences in cardiovascular response to stress* (pp. 125–145). New York: Plenum.

Anderson, N.B., Lane, J.D., Muranaka, H., Williams, R.B., Jr., & Houseworth, S.A. (1988). Racial differences in cardiovascular reactivity to mental arithmetic. *International Journal of Psychophysiology, 6*, 161–164.

Andreassi, J.L. (1989). *Psychophysiology: Human behavior and physiological response* (2nd ed.). Hillsdale, NJ: Erlbaum.

Arena, J.G., Blanchard, E.B., Andrasik, F., Cotch, P.A., & Myers, P.E. (1983). Reliability of psychophysiological assessment. *Behavior and Research Therapy, 21*, 447–460.

Armstrong, H.G., & Rafferty, J.A. (1950).Cold pressor test follow-up study for seven years on 166 officers. *American Heart Journal, 39*, 484–490.

Astrand, P.O., & Rodahl, K. (1977). *Textbook of work physiology* (2nd ed.). New York: McGraw-Hill.

Atlas, S.A., Sealey, J.E., & Laragh, J.H. (1989). The renin-angiotensin-aldosterone system and atrial natriuretic factor. In N. Schneiderman, S.M. Weiss, & P.G. Kaufmann (Eds.), *Handbook of research methods in cardiovascular behavioral medicine* (pp. 237–257). New York: Plenum.

Bahrke, M.S., & Morgan, W.P. (1978). Anxiety reduction following exercise and meditation. *Cognitive Research and Therapy, 2*, 323–333.

Bendig, A.W. (1956). The development of a short form of the Manifest Anxiety Scale. *Journal of Consulting Psychology, 20*, 384.

Berger, B.G., & Owen, D.R. (1988). Stress reduction and mood enhancement in four exercise modes: Swimming, body conditioning, Hatha yoga, and fencing. *Research Quarterly in Exercise and Sport, 59*, 148–159.

Berne, R.M., & Levy, M.N. (1986). *Cardiovascular physiology* (5th ed.). St. Louis: Mosby.

Bernstein, D.A., Roy, E.J., Srull, T.K., & Wickens, C.D. (1991). *Psychology* (2nd ed.). Boston: Houghton Mifflin.

Berntson, G.G., Cacioppo, J.T., & Quigley, K.S. (1991). Autonomic determinism: The modes of autonomic control, the doctrine of autonomic space, and the laws of autonomic constraint. *Psychological Reviews, 98*, 459–487.

Berntson, G.G., Cacioppo, J.T., & Quigley, K.S. (1993). Respiratory sinus arrhythmia: Autonomic origins, physiological mechanism, and psychophysiological implications. *Psychophysiology, 30*, 183–196.

Bezucha, G.R., Lenser, M.C., Hanson,P.G., & Nagle, F.J. (1982). Comparison of hemodynamic responses to static and dynamic exercise. *Journal of Applied Physiology, 53*, 1589–1593.

Birk, L. (1973). *Biofeedback: Behavioral medicine.* New York: Grune & Stratton.

Blix, A.S., Stromme, S.B., & Ursin, H. (1974). Additional heart rate—An indicator of psychological activation. *Aerospace Medicine, 45*, 1219–1222.

Blumenthal, J.A., Emery, C.F., Walsh, M.A., Cox, D.R., Kuhn, C.M., Williams, R.B., Jr., & Williams, R.S. (1988). Exercise training in healthy Type A middle-aged men: Effects on behavioral and cardiovascular responses. *Psychosomatic Medicine, 50*, 418–433.

Blumenthal, J.A., Fredrikson, M., Kuhn, C.M., Ulmer, R.A., Walsh-Riddle, M., &

Appelbaum, M. (1990). Aerobic exercise reduces levels of cardiovascular and sympathoadrenal responses to mental stress in subjects without prior evidence of myocardial ischemia. *American Journal of Cardiology, 65,* 93–98.

Boomsma, D.I., & Gabrielli, W.F., Jr. (1985). Behavioral genetic approaches to psychophysiological data. *Psychophysiology, 22,* 249–260.

Borghi, C., Costa, F., Boschi, S., Mussi, A., & Ambrosioni, E. (1986). Predictors of stable hypertension in young borderline subjects: A five-year follow-up study. *Journal of Cardiovascular Pharmacology, 8* (Suppl. 5), S138–S141.

Bosimini, E., Galli, M., Guagliumi, G., Giubbini, R., & Tavazzi, L. (1991). Electrographic markers of ischemia during mental stress testing in postinfarction patients: Role of body surface mapping. *Circulation, 83* (Suppl. II), II-115–II-127.

Brantley, J., Dietz, L., McKnight, G., Jones, G., & Tulley, R. (1988). Convergence between the daily stress inventory: Validity and endocrine measures of stress. *Journal of Consulting and Clinical Psychology, 56,* 549.

Brener, J. (1967). Heart rate. In P.H. Venables & I. Martin (Eds.), *A manual of psychophysiological methods.* Amsterdam: North Holland.

Brod, J., Fencl, V., Hejl, Z., & Jirka, J. (1959). Circulatory changes underlying blood pressure elevation during acute emotional stress (mental arithmetic) in normotensive and hypertensive subjects. *Clinical Science, 18,* 269–279.

Cannon, W.B. (1927). The James-Lange theory of emotions: A critical examination and an alternative. *American Journal of Psychology, 39,* 106–124.

Cannon, W.B. (1929). *Bodily changes in pain, hunger, fear, and rage* (2nd ed.). New York: Appleton.

Cannon, W.B. (1935). Stresses and strains of homeostasis (Mary Scott Newbold lecture). *American Journal of Medical Sciences, 189,* 1–14.

Carmelli, D., Swan, G.E., Robinette, D., & Fabsitz, R. (1992). Genetic influence on smoking: A study of male twins. *New England Journal of Medicine, 327,* 829–833.

Carroll, D. (1984). *Biofeedback in practice.* New York: Longman.

Carroll, D. (1992). *Health psychology: Stress, behaviour and disease.* London: The Falmer Press.

Carroll, D., Turner, J.R., Lee, H.J., & Stephenson, J. (1984). Temporal consistency of individual differences in cardiac response to a video game. *Biological Psychology, 19,* 81–93.

Carroll, D., Hewitt, J.K., Last, K.A., Turner, J.R., & Sims, J. (1985). A twin study of cardiac reactivity and its relationship to parental blood pressure. *Physiology and Behavior, 34,* 103–106.

Carroll, D., Turner, J.R., & Hellawell, J.C. (1986a). Heart rate and oxygen consumption during active psychological challenge: The effects of level of difficulty. *Psychophysiology, 23,* 174–181.

Carroll, D., Turner, J.R., & Prasad, R. (1986b). The effects of level of difficulty of mental arithmetic challenge on heart rate and oxygen consumption. *International Journal of Psychophysiology, 4,* 167–173.

Carroll, D., Turner, J.R., & Rogers, S. (1987). Heart rate and oxygen consumption during mental arithmetic, a video game, and graded static exercise. *Psychophysiology, 24,* 112–118.

Carroll, D., Cross, G., & Harris, M.G. (1990). Physiological activity during a prolonged mental stress test: Evidence for a shift in the control of pressor reactions. *Journal of Psychophysiology, 4,* 261–269.

Carroll, D., Harris, M.G., & Cross, G. (1991). Haemodynamic adjustments to mental stress in normotensives and subjects with mildly elevated blood pressure. *Psychophysiology, 28*, 439–447.

Chapleau, M.W., Hajduczok, G., & Abboud, F.M. (1989). Peripheral and central mechanisms of baroreflex resetting. *Clinical and Experimental Pharmacology and Physiology, 15* (Suppl.), 31–43.

Chesney, M.A., & Ironson, G.H. (1989). Diaries in ambulatory monitoring. In N. Schneiderman, S.M., Weiss, & P.G. Kaufmann (Eds.), *Handbook of research methods in cardiovascular behavioral medicine* (pp. 317–331). New York: Plenum.

Chubon, R.A. (1987). Development of a quality-of-life rating scale for use in health care evaluation. *Evaluation and the Health Professions, 10*, 186–200.

Cohen, S., & Syme, L.S. (1985). *Social support and health.* New York: Academic Press.

Coleman, T.G., Granger, H.J., & Guyton, A.C. (1971). Whole-body circulatory autoregulation and hypertension. *Circulation Research, 29* (Suppl. 2), 1176–1186.

Cook, W.W., & Medley, D.M. (1954). Proposed hostility and pharisaic-virtue scales for the MMPI. *Journal of Applied Psychology, 38*, 414–418.

Cox, J.P., Evans, J.F., & Jamieson, J.L. (1979). Aerobic power and tonic heart rate responses to psychological stressors. *Personality and Social Psychology Bulletin, 5*, 160–163.

Crowne, D.P., & Marlowe, D. (1964). *The approval motive: Studies in evaluative dependence.* New York: Wiley.

Dawkins, R. (1989). *The selfish gene* (2nd ed.). New York: Oxford University Press.

Dembroski, T.M., & Costa, P.T., Jr. (1988). Assessment of coronary-prone behavior: A current overview. *Annals of Behavioral Medicine, 10*, 60–63.

Dembroski, T.M., MacDougall, J.M., Slaats, S., Eliot, R.S., & Buell, J.C. (1981). Challenge-induced cardiovascular response as a predictor of minor illnesses. *Journal of Human Stress, 7*, 2–5.

de Geus, E.J.C., van Doornen, L.J.P., de Visser, D.C., & Orlebeke, J.F. (1990). Existing and training induced differences in aerobic fitness: Their relationship to physiological response patterns during different types of stress. *Psychophysiology, 27*, 457–478.

DeQuattro, V., & Lee, D.D.-P. (1991). Blood pressure reactivity and sympathetic hyperactivity: Predictors of hypertension. *American Journal of Hypertension, 4*, 624S–628S.

Devereux, R.B., Pickering, T.G., Harshfield, G.A., Kleinert, H.D., Denby, L., Clark, L., Pregibon, D., Jason, M., Kleiner, B., Borer, J.S., & Laragh, J.H. (1983). Left ventricular hypertrophy in patients with hypertension: Importance of blood pressure response to regularly occurring stress. *Circulation, 68*, 470–476.

Dimsdale, J.E., & Ziegler, M.G. (1991). What do plasma and urinary measures of catecholamines tell us about human response to stressors? *Circulation, 83* (Suppl. II), II-36–II-42.

Ditto, B. (1993). Familial influences on heart rate, blood pressure, and self-report anxiety responses to stress: Results from 100 twin pairs. *Psychophysiology*, in press.

Drummond, P.D. (1983). Cardiovascular reactivity in mild hypertension. *Journal of Psychosomatic Research, 27*, 291–297.

Durel, L.A., Kus, L.A., Anderson, N.B., McNeilly, M., Llabre, M.M., Spitzer, S., Saab, P.G., Efland, J., Williams, R., & Schneiderman, N. (1993). Patterns and stability of cardiovascular responses to variations of the cold pressor test. *Psychophysiology, 30*, 39–46.

Eaves, L.J., Last, K.A., Young, P.A., & Martin, N.G. (1978). Model-fitting approaches to the analysis of human behaviour. *Heredity, 41*, 249–320.

Epstein, F.H., & Eckoff, R.D. (1967). The epidemiology of high blood pressure—Geographic distributions and etiological factors. In J. Stamler, R. Stamler, & T.N. Pullman (Eds.), *The epidemiology of hypertension* (pp. 155–166). New York: Grune & Stratton.

Ewart, C.K., & Kolodner, K.B. (1991). Social competence interview for assessing physiological reactivity in adolescents. *Psychosomatic Medicine, 53*, 289–304.

Ewart, C.K., & Kolodner, K.B. (1993). Predicting ambulatory blood pressure during school: Effectiveness of social and nonsocial reactivity tasks in black and white adolescents. *Psychophysiology, 30*, 30–38.

Fabsitz, R.R., Carmelli, D., & Hewitt, J.K. (1992). Evidence for independent genetic influences on obesity in middle age. *International Journal of Obesity, 16*, 657–666.

Fahrenberg, J., Schneider, H.-J., Foerster, F., Myrtek, M., & Muller, W. (1985). The quantification of cardiovascular reactivity in longitudinal studies. In A. Steptoe, H. Rüddel, & H. Neus (Eds.), *Clinical and methodological issues in cardiovascular psychophysiology* (pp. 107–120). Berlin: Springer-Verlag.

Falkner, B. (1989). Measurement of volume regulation: Renal function. In N. Schneiderman, S.M. Weiss, & P.G. Kaufmann (Eds.), *Handbook of research methods in cardiovascular behavioral medicine* (pp. 117–129). New York: Plenum.

Falkner, B., & Light, K.C. (1986). The interactive effects of stress and dietary sodium on cardiovascular reactivity. In K.A. Matthews, S.M. Weiss, T. Detre, T.M. Dembroski, B. Falkner, S.B. Manuck, & R.B. Williams, Jr. (Eds.), *Handbook of stress, reactivity, and cardiovascular disease* (pp. 329–341). New York: Wiley.

Falkner, B., Kushner, H., Onesti, G., & Angelakos, E.T. (1981). Cardiovascular characteristics in adolescents who develop essential hypertension. *Hypertension, 3*, 521–527.

Feinleib, M. (1979). Genetics and familial aggregation of blood pressure. In G. Onesti & C.R. Klimt (Eds.), *Hypertension: Determinants, complications and intervention* (pp. 35–48). New York: Grune & Stratton.

Feinleib, M., Garrison, R., Borhani, N., Rosenman, R., & Christian, J. (1975). Studies of hypertension in twins. In O. Paul (Ed.), *Epidemiology and control of hypertension* (pp. 3–20). New York: Stratton Intercontinental Medical Book Corporation.

Fillingim, R.B., & Blumenthal, J.A. (1992). Does aerobic fitness reduce stress responses? In J.R. Turner, A. Sherwood, & K.C. Light (Eds.), *Individual differences in cardiovascular response to stress* (pp. 203–217). New York: Plenum.

Flamenbaum, W., Weber, M.A., McMahon, G., Materson, B., Albert, A., & Poland, M. (1985). Monotherapy with labetolol compared with propranolol: Differential effects by race. *Journal of Clinical Hypertension, 75*, 24–31.

Folkman, S., & Lazarus, R.S. (1980). An analysis of coping in a middle-aged community sample. *Journal of Health and Social Behavior, 21*, 219–239.

Folkow, B. (1982). Physiological aspects of primary hypertension. *Physiological Reviews, 62*, 347–504.

Folkow, B. (1990). "Structural factor" in primary and secondary hypertension. *Hypertension, 16*, 89–101.

Folkow, B., and Neil, E. (1971). *Circulation*. New York: Oxford University Press.

Forsyth, R.P. (1971). Regional blood-flow changes during 72-hour avoidance schedules in the monkey. *Science, 173*, 546–548.

Frankenhaeuser, M. (1991). The psychophysiology of workload, stress, and health: Comparison between the sexes. *Annals of Behavioral Medicine, 13*, 197–204.

Fredrikson, M. (1986). Racial differences in reactivity to behavioral challenges in essential hypertension. *Journal of Hypertension, 4*, 325–331.

Fredrikson, M., & Matthews, K.A. (1990). Cardiovascular responses to behavioral stress and hypertension: A meta-analytic review. *Annals of Behavioral Medicine, 12*, 30–39.

Friedman, B.H., Thayer, J.F., Borkovec, T.D., Tyrrell, R.A., Johnsen, B-H., & Colombo, R. (1993). Autonomic characteristics of nonclinical panic and blood phobia. *Biological Psychiatry, 34*, 298–310.

Frohlich, E.D., Kozul, V.J., Tarazi, R.C., & Dustan, H.P. (1970). Physiological comparison of labile and essential hypertension. *Circulation Research, 27* (Suppl. I), 55–69.

Gardner, E. (1975). *Fundamentals of neurology* (6th ed.). Philadelphia: Saunders.

Gatchel, R.J., Baum, A., & Krantz, D.S. (1989). *An introduction to health psychology* (2nd ed.). New York: Random House.

Gellman, M., Spitzer, S., Ironson, G., Llabre, M., Saab, P., DeCarlo Pasin, R., Weidler, D.J., & Schneiderman, N. (1990). Posture, place, and mood effects on ambulatory blood pressure. *Psychophysiology, 27*, 544–551.

Gerin, W., Pieper, C., Levy, R., & Pickering, T.G. (1992). Social support in social interaction: A moderator of cardiovascular reactivity. *Psychosomatic Medicine, 54*, 324–336.

Girdler, S.S., Turner, J.R., Sherwood, A., & Light, K.C. (1990). Gender differences in blood pressure control during a variety of behavioral stressors. *Psychosomatic Medicine, 52*, 571–591.

Girdler, S.S., Hinderliter, A.L., & Light, K.C. (1992). Peripheral adrenergic receptor contributions to cardiovascular reactivity: Influence of race and gender. *Journal of Psychosomatic Research, 37*, 177–193.

Girdler, S.S., Pedersen, C.A., Stern, R.A., & Light, K.C. (1993). The menstrual cycle and premenstrual syndrome: Modifiers of cardiovascular reactivity in women. *Health Psychology, 12*, 180–192.

Glass, D.C., Krakoff, L.R., Contrada, R., Hilton, W.F., Kehoe, K., Mannucci, E.G., Collins, C., Snow, B., & Elting, E. (1980). Effect of harassment and competition upon cardiovascular and plasma catecholamine responses in type A and type B individuals. *Psychophysiology, 17*, 453–463.

Gliner, J.A., Bunnell, D.E., & Horvath, S.M. (1982). Hemodynamic and metabolic changes prior to speech performance. *Physiological Psychology, 10*, 108–113.

Goble, M.M., & Schieken, R.M. (1991). Blood pressure response to exercise: A marker for future hypertension? *American Journal of Hypertension, 4*, 617S–620S.

Goldwater, B.C., & Collis, M.L. (1985). Psychologic effects of cardiovascular conditioning: A controlled experiment. *Psychosomatic Medicine, 47*, 174–181.

Greenberg, J.S. (1993). *Comprehensive stress management*. Dubuque, IA: Wm. C. Brown.

Grignani, G., Soffiantino, F., Zucchella, M., Pacchiarini, L., Tacconi, F., Bonomi, E., Pastoris, A., Sbaffi, A., Fratino, P., & Tavazzi, L. (1991). Platelet activation by emotional stress in patients with coronary artery disease. *Circulation, 83* (Suppl. II), II-128–II-136.

Grossman, P. (1983). Respiration, stress, and cardiovascular function. *Psychophysiology, 20*, 284–300.

Grossman, P., & Wientjes, K. (1985). Respiratory-cardiac coordination as an index of cardiac functioning. In J.F. Orlebeke, G. Mulder, & L.J.P. van Doornen (Eds.), *Psychophysiology of cardiovascular control: Models, methods, and data* (pp. 451–464). New York: Plenum.

Grossman, P., Karemaker, J., & Wieling, W. (1991). Prediction of tonic parasympathetic control using respiratory sinus arrhythmia: The need for respiratory control. *Psychophysiology, 28*, 201–216.

Grossman, P., Brinkman, A., & deVries, J. (1992). Cardiac autonomic mechanisms associated with borderline hypertension under varying behavioral demands: Evidence for attenuated parasympathetic tone but not for enhanced beta-adrenergic activity. *Psychophysiology, 29*, 698–711.

Guyton, A.C. (1977a). *Basic human physiology*. Philadelphia: Saunders.

Guyton, A.C. (1977b). Personal views on mechanisms of hypertension. In J. Genest, E. Koiw, & O. Kuchel (Eds.), *Hypertension: Physiopathology and treatment*. New York: McGraw-Hill.

Guyton, A.C. (1981). *Textbook of medical physiology* (6th ed.). Philadelphia: Saunders.

Guyton, A.C. (1989). Dominant role of the kidneys and accessory role of whole-body autoregulation in the pathogenesis of hypertension. *American Journal of Hypertension, 2*, 575–585.

Guyton, A.C., Coleman, T.G., Bower, J.D., & Granger, H.J. (1970). Circulatory control in hypertension. *Circulation Research, 27* (Suppl. II), 135–148.

Harlan, W.R., Osborne, R.K., & Graybiel, A. (1964). Prognostic value of the cold pressor test and the basal blood pressure: Based on an eighteen-year follow-up study. *American Journal of Cardiology, 13*, 683–687.

Harshfield, G.A., & Pulliam, D.A. (1992). Individual differences in ambulatory blood pressure patterns. In J.R. Turner, A. Sherwood, & K.C. Light (Eds.), *Individual differences in cardiovascular response to stress* (pp. 51–61). New York: Plenum.

Hastrup, J.L. (1986). Duration of initial heart rate assessment in *Psychophysiology*: Current practices and implications. *Psychophysiology, 23*, 15–18.

Hastrup, J.L., Light, K.C., & Obrist, P.A. (1980). Relationship of cardiovascular stress response to parental history of hypertension and to sex differences. *Psychophysiology, 17*, 317–318 (Abstract).

Haynes, S.G., & Matthews, K.A. (1988). Review and methodologic critique of recent studies on type A behavior and cardiovascular disease. *Annals of Behavioral medicine, 10*, 47–59.

Heath, A.C., Neale, M.C., Hewitt, J.K., Eaves, L.J., & Fulker, D.W. (1989). Testing structural equation models for twin data using LISREL. *Behavior Genetics, 19*, 9–35.

Heath, A.C., Meyer, J., Jardine, R., & Martin, N.G. (1991). The inheritance of alcohol consumption patterns in a general population twin sample: II. Determinants of consumption frequency and quantity consumed. *Journal of Studies on Alcohol, 52*, 425–433.

Hewitt, J.K., Stunkard, A.J., Carroll, D., Sims, J., & Turner, J.R. (1991). A twin study approach towards understanding genetic contributions to body size and metabolic rate. *Acta Geneticae Medicae et Gemellalogiae, 40*, 133–146.

Hinderliter, A.L., Light, K.C., & Willis, P.W., IV. (1991). Left ventricular mass index and diastolic filling: Relation to blood pressure and demographic variables in a healthy biracial sample. *American Journal of Hypertension, 4*, 479–585.

Hines, E.A., Jr. (1940). Significance of vascular hyperreaction as measured by the cold pressor test. *American Heart Journal, 19*, 408–416.

Hollander, B.J., & Seraganian, P. (1984). Aerobic fitness and psychophysiological reactivity. *Canadian Journal of Behavioral Science, 16*, 257–261.

Hollandsworth, J.G., Jr. (1986). *Physiology and behavior therapy: Conceptual guidelines for the clinician*. New York: Plenum.

Holmes, D.S., & Roth, D.L. (1985). Association of aerobic fitness with pulse rate and subjective responses to psychological stress. *Psychophysiology, 22*, 525–529.

Holmes, T.H., & Rahe, R.H. (1967). The social readjustment rating scale. *Journal of Psychosomatic Research, 14*, 121–132.

House, J.S., Landis, K.R., & Umberson, D. (1988). Social relationships and health. *Science, 241*, 540–545.

Houston, B.K. (1972). Control over stress, locus of control, and response to stress. *Journal of Personality and Social Psychology, 21*, 249–255.

Houston, B.K. (1989). Personality dimensions in reactivity and cardiovascular disease. In N. Schneiderman, S.M. Weiss, & P.G. Kaufmann (Eds.), *Handbook of research methods in cardiovascular behavioral medicine* (pp. 495–509). New York: Plenum.

Houston, B.K. (1992). Personality characteristics, reactivity, and cardiovascular disease. In J.R. Turner, A. Sherwood, & K.C. Light (Eds.), *Individual differences in cardiovascular response to stress* (pp. 103–123). New York: Plenum.

Hull, E.M., Young, S.H., & Ziegler, M.G. (1984). Aerobic fitness affects cardiovascular and catecholamine responses to stressors. *Psychophysiology, 21*, 353–360.

Hunt, S.C., Hasstedt, S.J., Kuida, H., Stults, B.M., Hopkins, P.N., & Williams, R.R. (1989). Genetic heritability and common environmental components of resting and stressed blood pressures, lipids, and body mass index in Utah pedigrees and twins. *American Journal of Epidemiology, 129*, 625–638.

Hunt, S.C., Williams, R.R., & Barlow, G.K. (1986). A comparison of positive family history definitions for defining risk of future disease. *Journal of Chronic Diseases, 39*, 809–821.

Hurwitz, B.E., Lu, C-C., Reddy, S.P., Shyu, L-Y., Schneiderman, N., & Nagel, J.H. (1993). Signal fidelity requirements for deriving impedance cardiographic measures of cardiac function over a broad range of heart rate. *Biological Psychology, 36*, 3–21.

Hurwitz, B.E., Shyu, L.-Y., Reddy, S.P., Schneiderman, N., & Nagel, J.H. (1990). Coherent ensemble averaging techniques for impedance cardiography. In H.T. Nagle & J.N. Brown (Eds.), *Computer-based medical systems* (pp. 228–235). Washington, DC: IEEE Computer Society Press.

Insel, P.A., & Motulsky, H.J. (1987). *Adrenergic receptors in man*. New York: Raven Press.

Ironson, G.H., Gellman, M.D., Spitzer, S.B., Llabre, M.M., DeCarlo Pasin, R., Weidler, D.J., & Schneiderman, N. (1989). Predicting home and work blood pressure measurements from resting baselines and laboratory reactivity in black and white Americans. *Psychophysiology, 26*, 174–184.

Jacob, R.G., & Chesney, M.A. (1986). Psychological and behavioral methods to reduce cardiovascular reactivity. In K.A. Matthews, S.M. Weiss, T. Detre, T.M. Dembroski, B. Falkner, S.B. Manuck, & R.B. Williams, Jr. (Eds.), *Handbook of stress, reactivity and cardiovascular disease* (pp. 417–457). New York: Wiley.

Jacob, R.G., Chesney, M.A., Williams, D.M., Ding, Y., & Shapiro, A.P. (1991). Relaxation therapy for hypertension: Design effects and treatment effects. *Annals of Behavioral Medicine, 13*, 5–17.

Jacobson, E. (1938). *Progressive relaxation*. Chicago: University of Chicago Press.

James, G.D., Pickering, T.G., Yee, L.S., Harshfield, G.A., Riva, S., & Laragh, J.H. (1988). The reproducibility of average ambulatory, home, and clinic pressures. *Hypertension, 11*, 545–549.

Jamieson, J.L., & Lavoie, N.P. (1987). Type A behavior, aerobic power and cardiovascular recovery from a psychosocial stressor. *Health Psychology, 6,* 361–371.

Jamner, L.D., Schwartz, G.E., & Leigh, H. (1988). The relationship between repressive and defensive coping styles and monocyte, eosinophile, and serum glucose levels: Support for the opioid peptide hypothesis of repression. *Psychosomatic Medicine, 50,* 567–575.

Jeffrey, R.W. (1991). Weight management and hypertension. *Annals of Behavioral Medicine, 13,* 18–22.

Jemerin, J.M., & Boyce, W.T. (1990). Psychobiological differences in childhood stress response: II. Cardiovascular markers of vulnerability. *Journal of Developmental and Behavioral Pediatrics, 11,* 140–150.

Jinks, J.L., & Fulker, D.W. (1970). Comparison of the biometrical genetical, MAVA, and classical approaches to the analysis of human behavior. *Psychological Bulletin, 73,* 311–349.

Johnston, D.W. (1989). Prevention of cardiovascular disease by psychological methods. *British Journal of Psychiatry, 154,* 183–194.

Johnston, D.W. (1992). The management of stress in the prevention of coronary heart disease. In S. Maes, H. Leventhal, & M. Johnston (Eds.), *International review of health psychology* (pp. 57–83). New York: Wiley.

Johnston, D.W., Anastasiades, P., & Wood, C. (1990). The relationship between cardiovascular responses in the laboratory and in the field. *Psychophysiology, 27,* 34–44.

Johnston, D.W., Anastasiades, P., Vogele, C., Clark, D.M., Kitson, C., & Steptoe, A. (1992). The relationship between cardiovascular responses in the laboratory and in the field: The importance of active coping. In T.H. Schmidt, B.T. Engel, & G. Blumchen (Eds.), *Temporal variations of the cardiovascular system* (pp. 127–144). Berlin: Springer-Verlag.

Jorde, L.B., & Williams, R.R. (1986). Innovative blood pressure measurements yield information not reflected by sitting measurements. *Hypertension, 8,* 252–257.

Jorgensen, R.S., & Houston, B.K. (1981). Family history of hypertension, gender, and cardiovascular reactivity and stereotypy during stress. *Journal of Behavioral Medicine, 4,* 175–189.

Julius, S. (1977a). Borderline hypertension: Epidemiologic and clinical implications. In J. Genest, E. Koiw, & O. Kuchel (Eds.), *Hypertension: Physiopathology and treatment* (pp. 630–640). New York: McGraw-Hill.

Julius, S. (1977b). Classification of hypertension. In J. Genest, E. Koiw, & O. Kuchel (Eds.), *Hypertension: Physiopathology and treatment* (pp. 9–12). New York: McGraw-Hill.

Julius, S. (1986). The emerging field of borderline hypertension. *Journal of Cardiovascular Pharmacology, 8,* 54–57.

Julius, S., & Esler, M. (1975). Autonomic nervous cardiovascular regulation in borderline hypertension. *American Journal of Cardiology, 36,* 685–696.

Julius, S., Randall, O.S., Esler, M.D., Kashima, T., Ellis, C., & Bennett, J. (1975). Altered cardiac responsiveness and regulation in the normal cardiac output type of borderline hypertension. *Circulation Research, 36–37(I),* I199–I207.

Kamarck, T.W., Manuck, S.B., & Jennings, J.R. (1990). Social support reduces cardiovascular reactivity to psychological challenge: A laboratory model. *Psychosomatic Medicine, 52,* 42–58.

Kamarck, T.W., Jennings, J.R., Debski, T.T., Glickman-Weiss, E., Johnson, P.S., Eddy, M.J., & Manuck, S.B. (1992). Reliable measures of behaviorally-evoked cardiovascular reactivity from a PC-based test battery: Results from student and community samples. *Psychophysiology, 29,* 17–28.

Kannel, W.B. (1979). The epidemiologic significance of familial and genetic factors in hypertension. In G. Onesti & C. R. Klimt (Eds.), *Hypertension: Determinants, complications, and intervention* (pp. 49–57). New York: Grune & Stratton.

Kannel, W.B., & Sorlie, P. (1975). Hypertension in Framingham. In O. Paul (Ed.), *Epidemiology and control of hypertension* (pp. 553–592). New York: Grune & Stratton, Intercontinental Medical Book Corporation.

Kannel, W.B., & Sorlie, P. (1979). Some health benefits of physical exercise: The Framingham study. *Archives of Internal Medicine, 139,* 857–861.

Kannel, W.B., & Thom, T.J. (1986). Incidence, prevalence and mortality of cardiovascular diseases. In J.W. Hurst (Ed.), *The heart, arteries and veins* (6th ed.) (pp. 557–565). New York: Plenum.

Kaplan, J.R., Manuck, S.B,. & Adams, M.R. (1991). Nonhuman primates as a model for evaluating behavioral influences on atherosclerosis, and cardiac structure and function. In A.P. Shapiro & A. Baum (Eds.), *Perspectives in behavioral medicine: Behavioral aspects of cardiovascular disease* (pp. 131–141). Hillsdale, NJ: Erlbaum.

Karasek, R.A., Theorell, T., Schwartz, J.E., Schnall, P.L., Pieper, C.F., & Michela, J.L. (1988). Job characteristics in relation to the prevalence of myocardial infarction in the U.S. Health Examination Survey (HES) and the Health and Nutrition Examination Survey (HANES). *American Journal of Public Health, 78,* 910–918.

Kasprowicz, A.L., Manuck, S.B., Malkoff, S.B., & Krantz, D.S. (1990). Individual differences in behaviorally evoked cardiovascular response: Temporal stability and hemodynamic patterning. *Psychophysiology, 27,* 605–619.

Kaufmann, P.G., Chesney, M.A., & Weiss, S.M. (1991). Behavioral medicine in hypertension: Time for new frontiers? *Annals of Behavioral Medicine, 13,* 3–4.

Kiecolt-Glaser, J.K., Cacioppo, J.T., Malarkey, W.B., & Glaser, R. (1992). Acute psychological stressors and short-term immune changes: What, why, for whom, and to what extent? *Psychosomatic Medicine, 54,* 680–685.

Klein, B. (1979). Genetics and familial aggregation of blood pressure. In G. Onesti & C.R. Klimt (Eds.), *Hypertension: Determinants, complications, and intervention* (pp. 59–62). New York: Grune & Stratton.

Krieger, E.M. (1989). Arterial baroreceptor resetting in hypertension. *Clinical and Experimental Pharmacology and Physiology, 15* (Suppl.), 3–17.

Lahey, B.B. (1992). *Psychology: An introduction* (4th ed.). Dubuque, IA: Wm. C. Brown.

Lane, J.D., Adcock, R.A., Williams, R.B., & Kuhn, C.M. (1990). Caffeine effects on cardiovascular and neuroendocrine responses to acute psychological stress and their relationship to level of habitual caffeine consumption. *Psychosomatic Medicine, 52,* 320–336.

Lane, J.D., Adcock, R.A., & Burnett, R.E. (1992). Respiratory sinus arrhythmia and cardiovascular responses to stress. *Psychophysiology, 29,* 461–470.

Langer, A.W., Obrist, P.A., & McCubbin, J.A. (1979). Hemodynamic and metabolic adjustments during exercise and shock avoidance in dogs. *American Journal of Physiology: Heart and Circulatory Physiology, 5,* H225–H230.

Langer, A.W., Hutcheson, J.S., Charlton, J.D., McCubbin, J.A., Obrist, P.A., & Stoney, C.M. (1985). On-line mini-computerized measurement of cardiopulmonary function on a breath-by-breath basis. *Psychophysiology, 25,* 50–58.

Langer, A.W., McCubbin, J.A., Stoney, C.M., Hutcheson, J.S., Charlton, J.D., & Obrist,

P.A. (1985). Cardiopulmonary adjustments during exercise and an aversive reaction time task: Effects of beta-adrenoceptor blockade. *Psychophysiology, 22,* 59–68.

Larkin, K.T., Manuck, S.B., & Kasprowicz, A.L. (1989). Heart rate feedback-assisted reduction in cardiovascular reactivity to a videogame challenge. *The Psychological Record, 39,* 365–371.

Larkin, K.T., Manuck, S.B., & Kasprowicz, A.L. (1990). The effect of feedback-assisted reduction in heart rate reactivity on videogame performance. *Biofeedback and Self-Regulation, 15,* 285–303.

Larkin, K.T., Zayfert, C., Abel, J.L., & Veltum, L.G. (1992a). Reducing heart rate reactivity to stress with feedback: Generalization across task and time. *Behavior Modification, 16,* 118–131.

Larkin, K.T., Zayfert, C., Veltum, L.G., & Abel, J.L. (1992b). Effects of feedback and contingent reinforcement in reducing heart rate responses to stress. *Journal of Psychophysiology, 6,* 119–130.

Larson, D.G., & Chastain, R.L. (1990). Self-concealment: Conceptualization, measurement and health implications. *Journal of Social and Clinical Psychology, 9,* 439–455.

Lawler, J.E., Barker, G.F., Hubbard, J.W., & Allen, M.T. (1980). The effects of conflict on tonic levels of blood pressure in the genetically borderline hypertensive rat. *Psychophysiology, 17,* 363–370.

Lawler, J.E., Barker, G.F., Hubbard, J.W., & Schaub, R.G. (1981). Effects of stress on blood pressure and cardiac pathology in rats with borderline hypertension. *Hypertension, 3,* 496–505.

Lazarus, R.S. (1966). *Psychological stress and the coping process.* New York: McGraw-Hill.

Lazarus, R.S., & Folkman, S. (1984). *Stress, appraisal and coping.* New York: Springer-Verlag.

Lazarus, R.S., & Launier, R. (1978). Stress-related transactions between person and environment. In L.A. Pervin & M. Lewis (Eds.), *Internal and external determinants of behavior.* New York: Plenum.

Lazarus, R.S., Opton, E.M., Jr., Nomikos, M.S., & Rankin, N.O. (1965). The principle of short-circuiting of threat: Further evidence. *Journal of Personality, 33,* 622–635.

Legato, M.J., & Colman, C. (1991). *The female heart: The truth about women and coronary artery disease.* New York: Simon & Schuster.

Lehrer, P.M., & Woolfolk, R.L. (1993). *Principles and practice of stress management* (2nd ed.). New York: Guilford.

Leon, A.S., Connett, J., Jacobs, D.R., & Rauramaa, R. (1987). Leisure-time physical activity levels and risk of coronary heart disease and death: The multiple risk factor intervention trial. *Journal of the American Medical Association, 258,* 2388–2395.

Levi, L. (1974). Psychosocial stress and disease: A conceptual model. In E.K.E. Gunderson & R.H. Rahe (Eds.), *Life stress and illness* (pp. 8–33). Springfield, IL: Charles C. Thomas.

Levy, R.L., White, P.D., Stroud, W.D., & Hillman, C.C. (1945). Transient hypertension. *Journal of the American Medical Association, 126,* 829–833.

Light, K.C. (1981). Cardiovascular responses to effortful active coping: Implications for the role of stress in hypertension development. *Psychophysiology, 18,* 216–225.

Light, K.C. (1989). Constitutional factors relating to differences in cardiovascular response. In N. Schneiderman, S.M. Weiss, & P.G.Kaufmann (Eds.), *Handbook of research methods in cardiovascular behavioral medicine* (pp. 417–431). New York: Plenum.

Light, K.C. (1992). Differential responses to salt-stress interactions: Relevance to hypertension. In J.R. Turner, A. Sherwood, & K.C. Light (Eds.), *Individual differences in cardiovascular response to stress* (pp. 245–263). New York: Plenum.

Light, K.C., & Sherwood, A. (1989). Race, borderline hypertension and hemodynamic responses to behavioral stress before and after beta-adrenergic blockade. *Health Psychology, 8,* 577–595.

Light, K.C., Koepke, J.P., Obrist, P.A., & Willis, P.W. (1983). Psychological stress induces sodium and fluid retention in men at high risk for hypertension. *Science, 220,* 429–431.

Light, K.C., Obrist, P.A., Sherwood, A., James, S., & Strogatz, D. (1987). Effects of race and marginally elevated blood pressure on cardiovascular responses to stress in young men. *Hypertension, 10,* 555–563.

Light, K.C., Obrist, P.A., & Cubeddu, L.X. (1988). Evaluation of a new ambulatory blood pressure monitor (Accutracker 102): Laboratory comparisons with direct arterial pressure, stethoscopic auscultatory pressure, and readings from a similar monitor (Spacelabs model 5200). *Psychophysiology, 25,* 107–116.

Light, K.C., Dolan, C.A., Davis, M.R., & Sherwood, A. (1992a). Cardiovascular responses to an active coping challenge as predictors of blood pressure patterns 10 to 15 years later. *Psychosomatic Medicine, 54,* 217–230.

Light, K.C., Sherwood, A., & Turner, J.R. (1992b). High cardiovascular reactivity to stress: A predictor of later hypertension development. In J.R. Turner, A. Sherwood, & K.C. Light (Eds.), *Individual differences in cardiovascular response to stress* (pp. 281–293). New York: Plenum.

Light, K.C., Turner, J.R., & Hinderliter, A.L. (1992c). Job strain and ambulatory blood pressure in healthy young men and women. *Hypertension, 20,* 214–218.

Light, K.C., Turner, J.R., Hinderliter, A., & Sherwood, A. (1993a). Race and gender comparisons: I. Hemodynamic responses to a series of stressors. *Health Psychology, 12,* 354–365.

Light, K.C., Turner, J.R., Hinderliter, A., & Sherwood, A. (1993b). Race and gender comparisons: II. Predictions of work blood pressure from laboratory baselines and cardiovascular reactivity measures. *Health Psychology, 12,* 366–375.

Llabre, M.M., Spitzer, S.B., Saab, P.G., Ironson, G.H., & Schneiderman, N. (1991). The reliability and specificity of delta versus residualized change as measures of cardiovascular reactivity to behavioral challenge. *Psychophysiology, 28,* 701–711.

Llabre, M.M., Saab, P.G., Hurwitz, B.E., Schneiderman, N., Frame, C.A., Spitzer, S., & Phillips, D. (1993). The stability of cardiovascular parameters under different behavioral challenges: One-year follow-up. *International Journal of Psychophysiology, 14,* 241–248.

Lovallo, W.R. (1975). The cold pressor test and autonomic function: A review and integration. *Psychophysiology, 12,* 268–282.

Lovallo, W.R., & Wilson, M.F. (1992a). A biobehavioral model of hypertension development. In J.R. Turner, A. Sherwood, & K.C. Light (Eds.), *Individual differences in cardiovascular response to stress* (pp. 265–280). New York: Plenum.

Lovallo, W.R., & Wilson, M.F. (1992b). The role of cardiovascular reactivity in hypertension risk. In J.R. Turner, A. Sherwood, & K.C. Light (Eds.), *Individual differences in cardiovascular response to stress* (pp. 165–186). New York: Plenum.

Lovallo, W.R., Wilson, M.F., Pincomb, G.A., Edwards, G.L., Tompkins, P., & Brackett, D.J. (1985). Activation patterns to aversive stimulation in man: Passive exposure versus effort to control. *Psychophysiology, 22,* 283–291.

Lovallo, W.R., Pincomb, G.A., & Wilson, M.F. (1986a). Heart rate reactivity and type A behavior as modifiers of physiological response to active and passive coping. *Psychophysiology, 23*, 105–112.

Lovallo, W.R., Pincomb, G.A., & Wilson, M.F. (1986b). Predicting response to a reaction time task: Heart rate reactivity compared with type A behavior. *Psychophysiology, 23*, 648–656.

Lund-Johansen, P. (1967). Haemodynamics in early essential hypertension. *Acta Medica Scandinavica* (Suppl. 182), 1–101.

Lund-Johansen, P. (1977). Central haemodynamics in essential hypertension. *Acta Medica Scandanavica* (Suppl. 606), 35–42.

Lund-Johansen, P. (1983). Hemodynamic alterations in early essential hypertension: Recent advances. In F. Gross & T. Strasser (Eds.), *Mild hypertension: Recent advances* (pp. 237–249). New York: Raven Press.

McArdle, W.D., Foglia, G.F., & Patti, A.V. (1967). Telemetered cardiac response to selected running events. *Journal of Applied Physiology, 23*, 566–570.

McCann, B.S., & Matthews, K.A. (1988). Influences of potential for hostility, Type A behavior, and parental history of hypertension on adolescents' cardiovascular responses during stress. *Psychophysiology, 25*, 503–511.

McCubbin, J.A., Cheung, R., Montgomery, T.B., Bulbulian, R., & Wilson, J.F. (1992). Endogenous opioids and stress reactivity in the development of essential hypertension. In J.R. Turner, A. Sherwood, & K.C. Light (Eds.), *Individual differences in cardiovascular response to stress* (pp. 221–243). New York: Plenum.

McCubbin, J.A., Kaplan, J.R., Manuck, S.B,. & Adams, M.R. (1993). Opioidergic inhibition of circulatory and endocrine stress responses in cynomolgus monkeys: A preliminary study. *Psychosomatic Medicine, 55*, 23–28.

McKinney, M.E., Miner, M.H., Ruddel, H., McIlvain, H.E., Witte, H., Buell, J.C., Eliot, R.S., & Grant, L.B. (1985). The standardized mental stress test protocol: Test-retest reliability and comparison with ambulatory blood pressure monitoring. *Psychophysiology, 22*, 453–463.

Mahoney, L.T., Clarke, W.R., Burns, T.L., & Lauer, R.M. (1991). Childhood predictors of high blood pressure. *American Journal of Hypertension, 4*, 608S–610S.

Mancia, G., Di Rienzo, M., & Parati, G. (1993). Ambulatory blood pressure monitoring use in hypertension research and clinical practice. *Hypertension, 21*, 510–524.

Manger, W.M. (1991). Obituary of Irvine Heinly Page, M.D. *Hypertension, 18* (Suppl. III), III-197–III-198.

Manuck, S.B., & Garland, F.N. (1980). Stability of individual differences in cardiovascular reactivity: A thirteen-month follow-up. *Physiology and Behavior, 24*, 621–624.

Manuck, S.B., & Krantz, D.S. (1986). Psychophysiologic reactivity in coronary heart disease and essential hypertension. In K.A. Matthews, S.M. Weiss, T. Detre, T.M. Dembroski, B. Falkner, S.B. Manuck, & R.B. Williams, Jr. (Eds.), *Handbook of stress, reactivity, and cardiovascular disease* (pp. 11–34). New York: Wiley.

Manuck, S.B., & Proietti, J.M. (1982). Parental hypertension and cardiovascular response to cognitive and isometric challenge. *Psychophysiology, 19*, 481–489.

Manuck, S.B., & Schaefer, D.C. (1978). Stability of individual differences in cardiovascular reactivity. *Physiology and Behavior, 21*, 675–678.

Manuck, S.B., Craft, S., & Gold, K.J. (1978). Coronary-prone behavior pattern and cardiovascular response. *Psychophysiology, 15*, 403–411.

222   REFERENCES

Manuck, S.B., Giordani, B., McQuaid, K.J., & Garrity, S.J. (1981). Behaviorally-induced cardiovascular reactivity among sons of reported hypertensive and normotensive parents. *Journal of Psychosomatic Research, 25*, 261–269.
Manuck, S.B., Kaplan, J.R., & Matthews, K.A. (1986). Behavioral antecedents of coronary heart disease and atherosclerosis. *Arteriosclerosis, 6*, 2–14.
Manuck, S.B., Kasprowicz, A.L., Monroe, S.M., Larkin, K.T., & Kaplan, J.R. (1989). Psychophysiological reactivity as a dimension of individual differences. In N. Schneiderman, S.M. Weiss, & P.G. Kaufmann (Eds.), *Handbook of research methods in cardiovascular behavioral medicine* (pp. 365–382). New York: Plenum.
Manuck, S.B., Kasprowicz, A.L., & Muldoon, M.F. (1990). Behaviorally-evoked cardiovascular reactivity and hypertension: Conceptual issues and potential associations. *Annals of Behavioral Medicine, 12*, 17–29.
Markovitz, J.H., & Matthews, K.A. (1991). Platelets and coronary heart disease: Potential psychophysiologic mechanisms. *Psychosomatic Medicine, 53*, 643–668.
Matarazzo, J.D. (1980). Behavioral health and behavioral medicine: Frontiers for a new health psychology. *American Psychologist, 35*, 807–817.
Matthews, K.A. (1992). Myths and realities of the menopause. *Psychosomatic Medicine, 54*, 1–9.
Matthews, K.A., & Rakaczky, C.J. (1986). Familial aspects of the type A behavior pattern and physiologic reactivity to stress. In T.H. Schmidt, T.M. Dembroski, & G. Blumchen (Eds.), *Biological and psychological factors in cardiovascular disease* (pp. 228–245). Berlin: Springer-Verlag.
Matthews, K.A., & Rodin, J. (1992). Pregnancy alters blood pressure responses to psychological and physical challenge. *Psychophysiology, 29*, 232–240.
Matthews, K.A., & Stoney, C.M. (1988). Influences of sex and age on cardiovascular responses during stress. *Psychosomatic Medicine, 50*, 46–56.
Matthews, K.A., Manuck, S.B., & Saab, P.G. (1986a). Cardiovascular responses of adolescents during a naturally occurring stressor and their behavioral and psychophysiological predictors. *Psychophysiology, 23*, 198–209.
Matthews, K.A., Weiss, S.M., Detre, T., Dembroski, T.M., Falkner, B., Manuck, S.B., & Williams, R.B., Jr. (1986b). *Handbook of stress, reactivity, and cardiovascular disease.* New York: Wiley.
Matthews, K.A., Rakaczky, C.J., Stoney, C.M., & Manuck, S.B. (1987). Are cardiovascular responses to behavioral stressors a stable individual difference variable in childhood? *Psychophysiology, 24*, 464–473.
Meichenbaum, D. (1985). *Stress inoculation training.* New York: Pergamon.
Meneely, G.R., & Battarbee, H.D. (1976). High sodium–low potassium environment and hypertension. *American Journal of Cardiology, 38*, 768–785.
Menkes, M.S., Matthews, K.A., Krantz, D.S., Lundberg, V., Mead, L.A., Qaqish, B., Liang, K.-Y., Thomas, C.B., & Pearson, T.A. (1989). Cardiovascular reactivity to the cold pressor test as a predictor of hypertension. *Hypertension, 14*, 524–530.
Miller, J.C., & Horvath, S.M. (1978). Impedance cardiography. *Psychophysiology, 15*, 80–91.
Miller, S.B. (1993). Parasympathetic nervous system control of heart rate responses to stress in offspring of hypertensives. *Psychophysiology,* in press.
Mills, P.J., & Dimsdale, J.E. (1988). The promise of receptor studies in psychophysiologic research. *Psychosomatic Medicine, 50*, 555–566.
Mills, P.J., & Dimsdale, J.E. (1991). Cardiovascular reactivity to psychosocial stressors: A review of the effects of beta-blockade. *Psychosomatics, 32*, 209–220.

Mills, P.J., & Dimsdale, J.E. (1992). Sympathetic nervous system responses to psychosocial stressors. In J.R. Turner, A. Sherwood, & K.C. Light (Eds.), *Individual differences in cardiovascular response to stress* (pp. 33–49). New York: Plenum.

Mills, P.J., & Dimsdale, J.E. (1993). The promise of receptor studies in psychophysiologic research: II. Applications, limitations, and progress. *Psychosomatic Medicine*, in press.

Morris, J.M., Everitt, M.G., Pollard, R., Chave, S.P.W., & Semmence, A.M. (1980). Vigorous exercise in leisure-time: Protection against coronary heart disease. *Lancet, 2*, 1207–1210.

Monroe, S.M. (1989). Stress and social support. In N. Schneiderman, S.M. Weiss, & P.G. Kaufmann (Eds.), *Handbook of research methods in cardiovascular behavioral medicine* (pp. 511–526). New York: Plenum.

Moses, J., Steptoe, A., Mathews, A., & Edwards, S. (1989). The effects of exercise training on mental well-being in the normal population: A controlled trial. *Journal of Psychosomatic Research, 33*, 47–61.

Muldoon, M.F., Terrell, D.F., Bunker, C.H., & Manuck, S.B. (1993). Family history studies in hypertension research: Review of the literature: *American Journal of Hypertension, 6*, 76–88.

Murphy, J.K. (1992). Psychophysiological responses to stress in children and adolescents. In P.M. La Greca, L.J. Siegal, J.L. Wallander, & C.E. Walker (Eds.), *Stress and coping in child health* (pp. 44–71). New York: Guilford.

Murphy, J.K., Alpert, B.S., Moes, D.M., & Somes, G.W. (1986). Race and cardiovascular reactivity: A neglected relationship. *Hypertension, 8*, 1075–1083.

Musante, L., Treiber, F.A., Strong, W.B., & Levy, M. (1990). Family history of hypertension and cardiovascular reactivity to forehead cold stimulation in black male children. *Journal of Psychosomatic Research, 34*, 111–116.

Myrtek, M. (1985). Adaptation effects and the stability of physiological responses to repeated testing. In A. Steptoe, H. Rüddel, & H. Neus (Eds.), *Clinical and methodological issues in cardiovascular psychophysiology* (pp. 93–106). Berlin: Springer-Verlag.

Nagel, J.H., Shyu, L-Y., Reddy, S.P., Hurwitz, B.E., McCabe, P.M., & Schneiderman, N. (1989). New signal processing techniques for improved precision of noninvasive impedance cardiography. *Annals of Biomedical Engineering, 17*, 517–534.

Nance, W.E. (1984). The relevance of twin studies in cardiovascular research. In D.C. Rao, R.C. Elston, & L.H. Kuller (Eds.), *Genetic epidemiology of coronary heart disease: Past, present, and future* (pp. 325–348). New York: Alan R. Liss.

Nestel, P.J. (1969). Blood pressure and catecholamine excretion after mental stress in labile hypertension. *Lancet, 1*, 692–694.

Norris, R., Carroll, D., & Cochrane, R. (1990). The effects of aerobic and anaerobic training on fitness, blood pressure, and psychological stress and well-being. *Journal of Psychosomatic Research, 34*, 367–375.

Norvell, N., & Belles, D. (1990). *Stress management training: A group leader's guide*. Sarasota, FL: Professional Resource Exchange.

Norvell, N., Roth, D.L., Franco, E., & Pepine, C.J. (1989). Cardiovascular reactivity and silent ischemia in response to mental stress in symptomatic and asymptomatic coronary artery disease patients: Results of a pilot study. *Clinical Cardiology, 12*, 634–638.

Obrist, P.A., (1976). The cardiovascular-behavioral interaction as it appears today. *Psychophysiology, 13*, 95–107.

Obrist, P.A. (1981). *Cardiovascular psychophysiology: A perspective*. New York: Plenum.

Obrist, P.A., & Light, K.C. (1988). Active-passive coping and cardiovascular reactivity: Interaction with individual differences and types of baseline. In W.A. Gordon, J.A.

Herd, & A. Baum (Eds.), *Perspectives on behavioral medicine* (Volume 3, pp. 109–126). San Diego: Academic Press.

Obrist, P.A., Langer, A.W., Light, K.C., & Koepke, J.P. (1983). Behavioral-cardiac interactions in hypertension. In D.S. Krantz, A. Baum, & J.E. Singer (Eds.), *Handbook of psychology and health: Vol. 3. Cardiovascular disorders and behavior* (pp. 199–230). Hillsdale, NJ: Erlbaum.

Obrist, P.A., Lawler, J.E., Howard, J.L., Smithson, K.W., Martin, P.L., & Manning, J. (1974). Sympathetic influences on cardiac rate and contractility during acute stress in humans. *Psychophysiology, 11*, 405–427.

Obrist, P.A., Gaebelein, C.J., Teller, S.E., Langer, A.W., Grignolo, A., Light, K.C., & McCubbin, J.A. (1978). The relationship among heart rate, carotid dP/dt and blood pressure in humans as a function of the type of stress. *Psychophysiology, 15*, 102–115.

Ornish, D. (1990). *Dr. Dean Ornish's program for reversing heart disease.* New York: Ballantine Books.

Ornstein, R., & Sobel, D.S. (1990). The brain as a health maintenance organization. In R. Ornstein & C. Swencionis (Eds.), *The healing brain: A scientific reader* (pp. 10–21). New York: Guilford.

Paffenbarger, R.S., Hale, W., Brand, R., & Hyde, B.J. (1977). Work-energy level, personal characteristics and fatal heart attack: A birth-cohort effect. *American Journal of Epidemiology, 105*, 200–213.

Paffenbarger, R.S., Hyde, R.T., Irving, A.S., & Steinmetz, C.H. (1984). A natural history of athleticism and cardiovascular health. *Journal of the American Medical Association, 252*, 491–495.

Page, I.H. (1977). Some regulatory mechanisms of renovascular and essential arterial hypertension. In J. Genest, E. Koiw, & O. Kuchel (Eds.), *Hypertension: Physiopathology and treatment* (pp. 576–587). New York: McGraw-Hill.

Parati, G., Pomidossi, G., Casadei, R., Ravogli, A., Groppelli, A., Cesana, B., & Mancia, G. (1988). Comparison of the cardiovascular effects of different laboratory stressors and their relationship with blood pressure variability. *Journal of Hypertension, 6*, 481–488.

Pattishall, E.G., Jr. (1989). The development of behavioral medicine: Historical models. *Annals of Behavioral Medicine, 11*, 43–48.

Paul, O. (1977). Epidemiology of hypertension. In J. Genest, E. Koiw, & O. Kuchel (Eds.), *Hypertension: Physiopathology and treatment* (p. 613–630). New York: McGraw-Hill.

Peckerman, A., Saab, P.G., McCabe, P.M., Skyler, J.S., Winters, R.W., Llabre, M.M., & Schneiderman, N. (1991). Blood pressure reactivity and the perception of pain during the forehead cold pressor test. *Psychophysiology, 28*, 485–495.

Perkins, K.A. (1989). Interactions among coronary heart disease risk factors. *Annals of Behavioral Medicine, 11*, 3–11.

Perloff, D., Sokolow, M., & Cowan, R. (1983). The prognostic value of ambulatory blood pressures. *Journal of the American Medical Association, 249*, 2793–2798.

Pescatello, L.S., Fargo, A.E., Leach, C.N., & Scherzer, H.H. (1991). Short-term effect of dynamic exercise on arterial blood pressure. *Circulation, 83*, 1557–1561.

Pickering, G. (1968). *High blood pressure* (2nd ed.). New York: Grune & Stratton.

Pickering, T.G. (1989). Ambulatory monitoring: Applications and limitations. In N. Schneiderman, S.M. Weiss, & P.G. Kaufmann (Eds.), *Handbook of research methods in cardiovascular behavioral medicine* (pp. 261–272). New York: Plenum.

Pickering, T.G. (1991a). *Ambulatory monitoring and blood pressure variability*. London: Science Press.

Pickering, T.G. (1991b). Challenge response predictors: General principles. *American Journal of Hypertension, 4*, 611S–614S.

Pickering, T.G., & Gerin, W. (1990). Cardiovascular reactivity in the laboratory and the role of behavioral factors in hypertension: A critical review. *Annals of Behavioral Medicine, 12*, 3–16.

Pickering, T.G., & Gerin, W. (1992). Does cardiovascular reactivity have pathogenic significance in hypertensive patients? In E.H. Johnson, W.D. Gentry, & S. Julius (Eds.), *Personality, elevated blood pressure, and essential hypertension* (pp. 151–173). Washington, DC: Hemisphere.

Pickering, T.G., James, G.D., Boddie, C., Harshfield, G.A., Blank, S., & Laragh, J.H. (1988). How common is white coat hypertension? *Journal of the American Medical Association, 259*, 225–228.

Pitts, R.F. (1974). *Physiology of the kidneys and body fluids* (3rd ed.). Chicago: Year Book Medical Publishers.

Plomin, R. (1990). The role of inheritance in behavior. *Science, 248*, 183–188.

Plomin, R., & Rende, R. (1991). Human behavioral genetics. *Annual Review of Psychology, 42*, 161–190.

Polefrone, J.M., & Manuck, S.B. (1988). Effects of menstrual phase and parental history of hypertension on cardiovascular response to cognitive challenge. *Psychosomatic Medicine, 50*, 23–36.

Porges, S.W. (1985). Respiratory sinus arrhythmia: An index of vagal tone. In J.F. Orlebeke, G. Mulder, & L.J.P. van Doornen (Eds.), *Psychophysiology of cardiovascular control: Models, methods, and data* (pp. 437–450). New York: Plenum.

Porges, S.W. (1986). Respiratory sinus arrhythmia: Physiological basis, quantitative methods, and clinical implications. In P. Grossman, K.H.L. Janssen, & D. Vaitl (Eds.), *Cardiorespiratory and cardiosomatic psychophysiology* (pp. 101–115). New York: Plenum.

Raven, J.C. (1960). *Guide to the standard progressive matrices*. London: H.K. Lewis.

Raven, J.C. (1962). *Guide to the advanced progressive matrices*. London: H.K. Lewis.

Rejeski, W.J., Thompson, A., Brubaker, P.H., & Miller, H.S. (1992). Acute exercise: Buffering psychosocial stress responses in women. *Health Psychology, 11*, 355–362.

Robertson, D., Parfyonova, Y., Menshikov, M., & Hollister, A.S. (1989). Receptors. In N. Schneiderman, S.M. Weiss, & P.G. Kaufmann (Eds.), *Handbook of research methods in cardiovascular behavioral medicine* (pp. 221 –236). New York: Plenum.

Rose, R.J. (1984). Familial influence on ambulatory blood pressure: Studies of normotensive twins. In M.A. Weber & J.I.M. Drayer (Eds.), *Ambulatory blood pressure monitoring* (pp. 167–172). New York: Springer-Verlag.

Rose, R.J. (1988). Genes, stress and the heart. *Stress Medicine, 4*, 265–271.

Rose, R.J. (1992). Genes, stress, and cardiovascular reactivity. In J.R. Turner, A. Sherwood, & K.C. Light (Eds.), *Individual differences in cardiovascular response to stress* (pp. 87–102). New York: Plenum.

Rose, R.J., & Chesney, M.A. (1986). Cardiovascular stress reactivity: A behavior-genetic perspective. *Behavior Therapy, 17*, 314–323.

Roskies, E., Seraganian, P., Oscasohn, R., Hanley, J.A., Collu, R., Martin, N., & Smilga, C. (1986). The Montreal type A intervention project: Major findings. *Health Psychology, 5*, 45–69.

Rotter, J. (1966). Generalized expectancies for internal versus external control of reinforcement. *Psychological Monographs, 80* (1, Whole No. 609).

Roy, M., & Steptoe, A. (1991). The inhibition of cardiovascular responses to mental stress following aerobic exercise. *Psychophysiology, 28,* 689–700.

Rushmer, R.F. (1976). *Cardiovascular dynamics* (4th ed.). Philadelphia: Saunders.

Rushmer, R.F. (1989). Structure and function of the cardiovascular system. In N. Schneiderman, S.M. Weiss, & P.G. Kaufmann (Eds.), *Handbook of research methods in cardiovascular behavioral medicine* (pp. 5–22). New York: Plenum.

Saab, P.G. (1989). Cardiovascular and neuroendocrine responses to challenge in males and females. In N. Schneiderman, S.M. Weiss, & P.G. Kaufmann (Eds.), *Handbook of research methods in cardiovascular behavioral medicine* (pp. 453–481). New York: Plenum.

Saab, P.G., Matthews, K.A., Stoney, C.M., & McDonald, R.H. (1989). Premenopausal and postmenopausal women differ in their cardiovascular and neuroendocrine responses to behavioral stressors. *Psychophysiology, 26,* 270–280.

Saab, P.G., Llabre, M.M., Hurwitz, B.E., Frame, C.A., Reineke, L.J., Fins, A.I., McCalla, J., Cieply, L.K., & Schneiderman, N. (1992). Myocardial and peripheral vascular responses to behavioral challenges and their stability in black and white Americans. *Psychophysiology, 29,* 384–397.

Saab, P.G., Llabre, M.M., Hurwitz, B.E., Schneiderman, N., Wohlgemuth, W., Durel, L.A., Massie, C., & Nagel, J. (1993). The cold pressor test: Vascular and myocardial response patterns and their stability. *Psychophysiology, 30,* 366–373.

Schieken, R.M., Clarke, W.R., & Lauer, R.M. (1981). Left ventricular hypertrophy in children with blood pressures in the upper quintile of the distribution: The Muscadine study. *Hypertension, 3,* 669–675.

Schieken, R.M., Eaves, L.J., Hewitt, J.K., Mosteller, M., Bodurtha, J.N., Moskowitz, W.B., & Nance, W.E. (1989). Univariate genetic analysis of blood pressure in children (the MCV Twin Study). *American Journal of Cardiology, 64,* 1333–1337.

Schnall, P.L., Pieper, C., Schwartz, J.E., Karasek, R.A., Schlussel, Y., Devereux, R.B., Ganau, A., Alderman, M., Warren, K., & Pickering, T.G. (1990). The relationship between "job strain," workplace diastolic blood pressure, and left ventricular mass index. *Journal of the American Medical Association, 263,* 1929–1935.

Schneiderman, N., & McCabe, P.M. (1989). Psychophysiological strategies in laboratory research. In N. Schneiderman, S.M. Weiss, & P.G. Kaufmann (Eds.), *Handbook of research methods in cardiovascular behavioral medicine* (pp. 349–364). New York: Plenum.

Schneiderman, N., Weiss, S.M., & Kaufmann, P.G. (1989). *Handbook of research methods in cardiovascular behavioral medicine.* New York: Plenum.

Schwartz, G.E., & Weiss, S.M. (1978). Behavioral medicine revisited: An amended definition. *Journal of Behavioral Medicine, 1,* 249–251.

Selye, H. (1956). *The stress of life.* New York: McGraw-Hill.

Selye, H. (1976). *The stress of life* (rev. ed.). New York: McGraw-Hill.

Shapiro, A.P., Krantz, D.S., & Grim, C.E. (1986). Pharmacologic agents as modulators of stress. In K.A. Matthews, S.M. Weiss, T. Detre, T.M. Dembroski, B. Falkner, S.B. Manuck, & R.B. Williams, Jr. (Eds.), *Handbook of stress, reactivity, and cardiovascular disease* (pp. 401–416). New York: Wiley.

Shapiro, A.P., Lane, J.D., & Henry, J.P. (1986). Caffeine, cardiovascular reactivity, and cardiovascular disease. In K.A. Matthews, S.M. Weiss, T. Detre, T.M. Dembroski, B. Falkner, S.B. Manuck, & R.B. Williams, Jr. (Eds.), *Handbook of stress, reactivity, and cardiovascular disease* (pp. 311–327). New York: Wiley.

Sherwood, A. (1993). Use of impedance cardiography in cardiovascular reactivity research. In J. Blascovich & E.S. Katkin (Eds.), *Cardiovascular reactivity to psychological stress and disease* (pp. 157–199). Washington, DC: American Psychological Association.

Sherwood, A., & Hinderliter, A.L. (1993). Responsiveness to α- and β-adrenergic receptor agonists: Effects of race in borderline hypertensive compared to normotensive men. *American Journal of Hypertension, 6,* 630–635.

Sherwood, A., & Turner, J.R. (1992). A conceptual and methodological overview of cardiovascular reactivity research. In J.R. Turner, A. Sherwood, & K.C. Light (Eds.), *Individual differences in cardiovascular response to stress* (pp. 3–32). New York: Plenum.

Sherwood, A., & Turner, J.R. (1993). Postural stability of hemodynamic responses during mental challenge. *Psychophysiology, 3,* 237–244.

Sherwood, A., Brener, J., & Moncur, D. (1983). Information and states of motor readiness: Their effects on the covariation of heart rate and energy expenditure. *Psychophysiology, 20,* 513–529.

Sherwood, A., Allen, M.T., Obrist, P.A., & Langer, A.W. (1986). Evaluation of beta-adrenergic influences on cardiovascular and metabolic adjustments to physical and psychological stress. *Psychophysiology, 23,* 89–104.

Sherwood, A., Light, K.C., & Blumenthal, J.A. (1989). Effects of aerobic exercise on hemodynamic responses during psychosocial stress in normotensive and borderline type A men: A preliminary report. *Psychosomatic Medicine, 51,* 123–136.

Sherwood, A., Allen, M.T., Fahrenberg, J., Kelsey, R.M., Lovallo, W.R., & van Doornen, L.J.P. (1990a). Committee report: Methodological guidelines for impedance cardiography. *Psychophysiology, 27,* 1–23.

Sherwood, A., Dolan, C.A., & Light, K.C. (1990b). Hemodynamics of blood pressure responses during active and passive coping. *Psychophysiology, 27,* 656–668.

Sherwood, A., Turner, J.R., Light, K.C., & Blumenthal, J.A. (1990c). Temporal stability of the hemodynamics of cardiovascular reactivity. *International Journal of Psychophysiology, 10,* 95–98.

Sherwood, A., Davis, M.R., Dolan, C.A., & Light, K.C. (1992a). Effects of self-challenge on cardiovascular reactivity. *International Journal of Psychophysiology, 12,* 87–94.

Sherwood, A., Royal, S.A., Hutcheson, J.S., & Turner, J.R. (1992b). Comparison of impedance cardiographic measurements using band and spot electrodes. *Psychophysiology, 29,* 734–741.

Sherwood, A., Royal, S.A., & Light, K.C. (1993). Laboratory reactivity assessment: Effects of casual blood pressure status and choice of task difficulty. *International Journal of Psychophysiology, 14,* 81–95.

Shumaker, S.A., & Czajkowski, S.M. (1992). *Social support and cardiovascular disease.* New York: Plenum.

Siegel, W.C., & Blumenthal, J.A. (1991). The role of exercise in the prevention and treatment of hypertension. *Annals of Behavioral Medicine, 13,* 23–30.

Sims, J., Hewitt, J.K., Kelly, K.A., Carroll, D., & Turner, J.R. (1986). Familial and individual influences on blood pressure. *Acta Geneticae Medicae et Gemellalogiae, 35,* 7–21.

Sims, J., Boomsma, D.I., Carroll, D., Hewitt, J.K., & Turner, J.R. (1991). Genetics of type A behavior in two European countries: Evidence for sibling interaction. *Behavior Genetics, 21,* 513–528.

Smith, M.A., & Houston, B.K. (1987). Hostility, anger expression, cardiovascular responsivity, and social support. *Biological Psychology, 24,* 39–48.

Smith, T.W. (1992). Hostility and health: Current status of a psychosomatic hypothesis. *Health Psychology, 11,* 139–150.

Smith, T.W., & Leon, A.S. (1992). *Coronary heart disease: A behavioral perspective.* Champaign, IL: Research Press.

Smith, T.W., Allred, K.D., Morrison, C.A., & Carlson, S.D. (1989). Cardiovascular reactivity and interpersonal influence: Active coping in a social context. *Journal of Personality and Social Psychology, 56,* 209–218.

Smith, T.W., Baldwin, M., & Christensen, A.J. (1990). Interpersonal influence as active coping: Effects of task difficulty on cardiovascular reactivity. *Psychophysiology, 27,* 429–437.

Smith, T.W., McGonigle, M., Turner, C.W., Ford, M.H., & Slattery, M.L. (1991). Cynical hostility in adult male twins. *Psychosomatic Medicine, 53,* 684–692.

Sparrow, D., Rosner, B., Vokonas, P.S., & Weiss, S.T. (1986). Relation of blood pressure measured in several positions to the subsequent development of systemic hypertension: The normative aging study. *American Journal of Cardiology, 57,* 218–221.

Spielberger, C.D., Jacobs, G., Russell, S., & Crane, R. (1983). Assessment of anger: The state-trait anger scale. In J.N. Butcher & C.D. Spielberger (Eds.), *Advances in personality assessment,* Vol. 2. Hillsdale, NJ: Erlbaum.

Spielberger, C.D., Johnson, E.H., Russell, S.F., Crane, R.J., Jacobs, G.A., & Worden, T.J. (1985). The experience and expression of anger: Construction and validation of an anger expression scale. In M.A. Chesney & R.H. Rosenman (Eds.), *Anger and hostility in cardiovascular and behavioral disorders* (pp. 5–30). New York: Hemisphere.

Stamler, R., Stamler, J., Riedlinger, W.F., Algera, G., & Roberts, R.H. (1971). Family (parental) history and prevalence of hypertension: Results of a nationwide screening program. *Journal of the American Medical Association, 241,* 43–46.

Steptoe, A. (1980). Blood pressure. In I. Martin & P.H. Venables (Eds.), *Techniques in psychophysiology* (pp. 247– 273). Chichester: Wiley.

Steptoe, A. (1981). *Psychological factors in cardiovascular disorders.* London: Academic Press.

Steptoe, A., & Bolton, J. (1988). The short-term influence of high and low intensity physical exercise on mood. *Psychology and Health, 2,* 91–106.

Steptoe, A., & Cox, S. (1988). Acute effects of aerobic exercise on mood. *Health Psychology, 7,* 329–340.

Steptoe, A., & Vögele, C. (1991). Methodology of mental stress testing in cardiovascular research. *Circulation, 83* (Suppl. II), II-14–II-24.

Steptoe, A., Melville, D., & Ross, A. (1984). Behavioral response demands, cardiovascular reactivity, and essential hypertension. *Psychosomatic Medicine, 46,* 33–48.

Steptoe, A., Edwards, S., Moses, J., & Mathews, A. (1989). The effects of exercise training on mood and perceived coping ability in anxious adults from the general population. *Journal of Psychosomatic Research, 33,* 537–547.

Stoney, C.M. (1992). The role of reproductive hormones in cardiovascular and neuroendocrine function during behavioral stress. In J.R. Turner, A. Sherwood, & K.C. Light (Eds.), *Individual differences in cardiovascular response to stress* (pp. 147–163). New York: Plenum.

Stoney, C.M., Davis, M.C., & Matthews, K.A. (1987). Sex differences in physiological responses to stress and in coronary heart disease: A causal link? *Psychophysiology, 24,* 127–131.

Stoney, C.M., Matthews, K.A., McDonald, R.H., & Johnson, C.A. (1988). Sex differences in lipid, lipoprotein, cardiovascular and neuroendocrine responses to acute stress. *Psychophysiology, 25,* 645–656.

Strogatz, D.S., & James, S.A. (1986). Social support and hypertension among blacks and whites in a rural, southern community. *American Journal of Epidemiology, 124,* 949–956.

Stromme, S.B., Wikeby, P.C., Blix, A.S., & Ursin, H. (1978). Additional heart rate. In H. Ursin, E. Baade, & S. Levine (Eds.), *Psychobiology of stress* (pp. 83–89). London: Academic Press.

Stunkard, A.J. (1991). Beginner's mind: Trying to learn something about obesity. *Annals of Behavioral Medicine, 13,* 51–56.

Stunkard, A.J., Foch, T.T., & Hrubec, Z. (1986). A twin study of human obesity. *Journal of the American Medical Association, 256,* 51–54.

Suarez, E.C., & Williams, R.B., Jr. (1989). Situational determinants of cardiovascular and emotional reactivity in high and low hostile men. *Psychosomatic Medicine, 51,* 404–418.

Suarez, E.C., & Williams, R.B., Jr. (1990). The relationships between dimensions of hostility and cardiovascular reactivity as a function of task characteristics. *Psychosomatic Medicine, 52,* 558–570.

Suarez, E.C., Williams, R.B., Jr., Kuhn, C.M., Zimmerman, E.H., & Schanberg, S.M. (1991). Biobehavioral basis of coronary-prone behavior in middle-aged men: Part II. Serum cholesterol, the type A behavior pattern and hostility as interactive modulators of physiological reactivity. *Psychosomatic Medicine, 53,* 528–537.

Surwit, R. (1986). Pharmacologic and behavioral modulators of cardiovascular reactivity: An overview. In K.A. Matthews, S.M. Weiss, T. Detre, T.M. Dembroski, B. Falkner, S.B. Manuck, & R.B. Williams, Jr. (Eds.), *Handbook of stress, reactivity, and cardiovascular disease* (pp. 385–400). New York: Wiley.

Tambs, K., Sundet, J.M., Eaves, L., & Berg, K. (1992). Genetic and environmental effects on type A scores in monozygotic twin families. *Behavior Genetics, 22,* 499–513.

Thomas, S.A., Lynch, J.J., Friedmann, E., Subinohara, M., Hall, P.S., & Peterson, C. (1984). Blood pressure and heart rate changes in children when they read aloud in school. *Public Health Reports, 99,* 77–84.

Treiber, F.A., Musante, L., Strong, W.B., & Levy, M. (1989). Racial differences in young children's blood pressure. *American Journal of Diseases in Children, 143,* 720–723.

Treiber, F.A., Musante, L., Braden, D., Arensman, F., Strong, W.B., Levy, M., & Leverett, S. (1990). Racial differences in hemodynamic responses to the cold face stimulus in children and adults. *Psychosomatic Medicine, 5,* 286–296.

Treiber, F.A., McCaffrey, F., Musante, L., Rhodes, T., Davis, H., Strong, W.B., & Levy, M. (1993). Ethnicity, family history of hypertension and patterns of hemodynamic reactivity in boys. *Psychosomatic Medicine, 55,* 70–77.

Turjanmaa, V. (1989). Determination of blood pressure level and changes in physiological situations: Comparison of the standard cuff method with direct intra-arterial recording. *Clinical Physiology, 9,* 373–387.

Turner, J.R. (1988). Inter-task consistency: An integrative review. *Psychophysiology, 25,* 235–238.

Turner, J.R. (1989). Individual differences in heart rate response during behavioral challenge. *Psychophysiology, 26,* 497–505.

Turner, J.R., & Carroll, D. (1985a). Heart rate and oxygen consumption during mental arithmetic, a video game, and graded exercise: Further evidence of metabolically-exaggerated cardiac adjustments? *Psychophysiology, 22,* 261–267.

Turner, J.R., & Carroll, D. (1985b). The relationship between laboratory and "real world" heart rate reactivity: An exploratory study. In J.F. Orlebeke, G. Mulder, & L.J.P. van Doornen

(Eds.), *Psychophysiology of cardiovascular control: Methods, models, and data* (pp. 895–907). New York: Plenum.

Turner, J.R., & Sherwood, A. (1991). Postural effects on blood pressure reactivity: Implications for studies of laboratory-field generalization. *Journal of Psychosomatic Research, 35,* 289–295.

Turner, J.R., & Hewitt, J.K. (1992). Twin studies of cardiovascular response to psychological challenge: A review and suggested future directions. *Annals of Behavioral Medicine, 14,* 12–20.

Turner, J.R., Carroll, D., & Courtney, H. (1983). Cardiac and metabolic responses to "space invaders": An instance of metabolically-exaggerated cardiac adjustment? *Psychophysiology, 20,* 544–549.

Turner, J.R., Carroll, D., Sims, J., Hewitt, J.K., & Kelly, K.A. (1986a). Temporal and inter-task consistency of heart rate reactivity during active psychological challenge: A twin study. *Physiology and Behavior, 38,* 641–644.

Turner, J.R., Hewitt, J.K., Morgan, R.K., Sims, J., Carroll, D., & Kelly, K.A. (1986b). Graded mental arithmetic as an active psychological challenge. *International Journal of Psychophysiology, 3,* 307–309.

Turner, J.R., Carroll, D., Dean, S., & Harris, M.G. (1987a). Heart rate reactions to standard laboratory challenges and a naturalistic stressor. *International Journal of Psychophysiology, 5,* 151–152.

Turner, J.R., Sims, J., Carroll, D., Morgan, R.K., & Hewitt, J.K. (1987b). A comparative evaluation of heart rate reactivity during MATH and a standard mental arithmetic task. *International Journal of Psychophysiology, 5,* 301–303.

Turner, J.R., Carroll, D., Costello, M., & Sims, J. (1988a). The effects of aerobic fitness on additional heart rates during active psychological challenge. *Journal of Psychophysiology, 2,* 91–97.

Turner, J.R., Carroll, D., Hanson, J., & Sims, J. (1988b). A comparison of additional heart rates during active psychological challenge calculated from upper body and lower body dynamic exercise. *Psychophysiology, 25,* 209–216.

Turner, J.R., Girdler, S.S., Sherwood, A., & Light, K.C. (1990). Cardiovascular responses to behavioral stressors: Laboratory-field generalization and inter-task consistency. *Journal of Psychosomatic Research, 34,* 581–589.

Turner, J.R., Sherwood, A., & Light, K.C. (1991). Generalization of cardiovascular response: Supportive evidence for the reactivity hypothesis. *International Journal of Psychophysiology, 11,* 207–212.

Turner, J.R., Sherwood, A., & Light, K.C. (1992). *Individual differences in cardiovascular response to stress.* New York: Plenum.

Turner, J.R., Cardon, L.R., & Hewitt, J.K. (1993a). *Behavioral genetic applications in behavioral medicine research.* New York: Plenum, *in press.*

Turner, J.R., Sherwood, A., & Light, K.C. (1993b). Intertask consistency of cardiovascular response in a biracial sample of men and women. Submitted.

Turner, J.R., Ward, M.M., Gellman, M.D., Johnston, D.W., Light, K.C., & van Doornen, L. J.P. (1993c). The relationship between laboratory and ambulatory cardiovascular activity: Current evidence and future directions. *Annals of Behavioral Medicine,* in press.

van Doornen, L.J.P., & de Geus, E.J.C. (1989). Aerobic fitness and the cardiovascular response to stress. *Psychophysiology, 26,* 17–28.

van Doornen, L.J.P., & Turner, J.R. (1992). The ecological validity of laboratory stress-testing. In J.R. Turner, A. Sherwood, & K.C. Light (Eds.), *Individual differences in cardiovascular response to stress* (pp. 63–83). New York: Plenum.

van Doornen, L.J.P., & van Blokland, R.W. (1992). The relationship between cardiovascular and catecholamine reactions to laboratory and real-life stress. *Psychophysiology, 29,* 173–181.

Van Egeren, L.F. (1992). Behavioral factors in blood pressure throughout the day: Effects of behavioral rhythms on blood pressure rhythms. In T.H. Schmidt, B.T. Engel, & G. Blumchen (Eds.), *Temporal variations of the cardiovascular system* (pp. 283–296). Berlin: Springer-Verlag.

Van Egeren, L.F., & Gellman, M.D. (1992). Cardiovascular reactivity to everyday events. In E.H. Johnson, W.D. Gentry, & S. Julius (Eds.), *Personality, elevated blood pressure, and hypertension* (pp. 135–150). Washington, DC: Hemisphere.

Van Egeren, L.F., & Madarasmi, S. (1988). A computer-assisted diary (CAD) for ambulatory blood pressure monitoring. *American Journal of Hypertension, 1,* 179s–185s.

Van Egeren, L.F., & Sparrow, A.W. (1989). Laboratory stress testing to assess real-life cardiovascular reactivity. *Psychosomatic Medicine, 51,* 1–9.

Vitaliano, P.P., Russo, J., Bailey, S.L., Young, H.M., & McCann, B.S. (1993). Psychosocial factors associated with cardiovascular reactivity in older adults. *Psychosomatic Medicine, 55,* 164–177.

von Eiff, A.W., Plotz, E.J., Beck, K.J., & Czernik, A. (1971). The effect of estrogens and progestins on blood pressure regulation of normotensive women. *American Journal of Obstetrics and Gynecology, 109,* 887–892.

Waldstein, S.R., Polefrone, J.M., Bachen, E.A., Muldoon, M.F., Kaplan, J.R., & Manuck, S.B. (1993). Relationship of cardiovascular reactivity and anger expression to serum lipid concentrations in healthy young men. *Journal of Psychosomatic Research, 37,* 249–256.

Weidner, G., Friend, R., Ficarrotto, T.J., & Mendell, N.R. (1989). Hostility and cardiovascular reactivity to stress in women and men. *Psychosomatic Medicine, 51,* 36–45.

Weinberger, D.A., Schwartz, G.E., & Davidson, R.J. (1979). Low-anxious, high-anxious, and repressive coping styles: Psychometric patterns and behavioral and physiological responses to stress. *Journal of Abnormal Psychology, 88,* 369–380.

Weiner, H. (1992). Specificity and specification: Two continuing problems in psychosomatic research. *Psychosomatic Medicine, 54,* 567–587.

Wilmore, J.H., & Norton, A.C. (1975). *The heart and lungs at work: A primer of exercise physiology.* Beckman Instruments Inc.

Wilson, M.F., Lovallo, W.R., & Pincomb, G.A. (1989). Noninvasive measurement of cardiac functions. In N. Schneiderman, S.M. Weiss, & P.G. Kaufmann (Eds.), *Handbook of research methods in cardiovascular behavioral medicine* (pp. 23–50). New York: Plenum.

Ziegler, M.G. (1989). Catecholamine measurement in behavioral research. In N. Schneiderman, S.M. Weiss, & P.G. Kaufmann (Eds.), *Handbook of research methods in cardiovascular behavioral medicine* (pp. 167–183). New York: Plenum.

Ziegler, M.G., Mills, P., & Dimsdale, J.E. (1991). Hypertensives' pressor response to norepinephrine: Analysis by infusion rate and plasma levels. *American Journal of Hypertension, 4,* 586–591.

Zuckerman, M., & Lubin, B. (1985). *Manual for the MAACL-R: The Multiple Affect Adjective Check List–Revised.* San Diego: Educational Testing Service.

Index

233